Dr. Earl Mindell's
NUTRITION
BIBLE

Dr. Earl Mindell's
NUTRITION
BIBLE

Dr. Earl Mindell & Virginia Hopkins

COUNCIL
OAK BOOKS

SAN FRANCISCO & TULSA

www.counciloakbooks.com

This revised and updated edition of *Earl Mindell's Nutrition Bible*
is based on *Earl Mindell's Diet Bible*, ©2002 by Earl Mindell, R.Ph.,
Ph.D. and One to One Inc., first published in the USA in 2003 by
Fair Winds Press, Gloucester, MA 01930

©2010, 2002 by Earl Mindell R.Ph., Ph.D. and One to One Inc.
First Council Oak Books edition, 2010. All rights reserved

BOOK AND COVER DESIGN: Carl Brune

COVER IMAGE: *Floating Fruit* © 2010 Otto Duecker.
Represented by Hammer Galleries, New York, NY;
M.A. Doran Gallery, Tulsa, OK; Llewellyn Gallery,
Santa Fe, NM; Robert Kidd Gallery, Birmingham, MI

First printing 2010

Printed in the USA

Library of Congress Cataloging in Publication data available

ISBN 978-1-57178-254-0

Dr. Earl Mindell would like to dedicate this book to: My wife and soul mate, Gail, to our children, Alanna and Evan, to all my friends and family for their support, and to the millions worldwide who now have a vehicle for winning the battle of the bulge without dieting or using any harmful substances.

Virginia Hopkins would like to dedicate this book to women and men who have struggled with weight issues.

TABLE OF CONTENTS

FACE IT, IF DIETS WORKED, obesity wouldn't be the number one health problem in Westernized countries. The Nutrition Bible is about learning how to fine-tune your miraculous body so that you're maintaining a healthy weight for optimal health and energy.

Instead of learning how to count calories and measure grams, you'll learn why food is your medicine, and why taking the pounds off and keeping them off isn't as much about staying away from calories as it is about moderation, balancing your blood sugar, and understanding what controls your appetite. You'll learn to choose the foods that work best for your body, and why you may want to shun health fads and eat more like your ancestors. I'm going to explain why insulin resistance and diabetes have reached epidemic levels in Westernized countries, how they develop, and why prescription drugs aren't the answer.

For centuries, Asians have used some amazing natural herbal secrets for weight loss. I'll reveal these to you. You'll discover how simple lifestyle changes can help you ramp up your energy and drop the pounds. And you'll learn about safe, effective nutrient supplements that work synergistically with your body's natural tendency towards healing and balance. Finally, I'll uncover what might be zapping your energy, and what it really means to exercise *your* body.

Nowhere in this book will you find instructions for exactly how much sugar, carbohydrate, fat, or protein you should eat. I'm not going to tell you to count calories, or eat certain percentages of fat. I will give you a few basic guidelines, but it's critical to your own personal success in achieving your optimal health and weight that you determine what works best for your body. The process of finding out what works for you will increase your awareness of why and how you eat, how it affects your energy, your ability to think clearly, your digestion, and over the long term, your weight. No diet will fit you for a lifetime unless it suits you perfectly, and the only diet that will work for you is one that you personally create over time.

Our goal in writing this book is to help you become more aware about how you interact with food, and how to use it to benefit your health, as well as to enhance your eating pleasure. It's up to you to use inherent common sense and discrimination to make better choices. For example, if you eat that chocolate volcano cake for dessert three times and then notice on the fourth time that you were irritable and craving sugar all the next day, then you have made progress. If you use that knowledge to eat less of it the fifth time or even eventually choose not to eat it, you are continuing to make progress. But you have not "lost" if you eat it again the seventh or tenth time and end up with a sugar hangover—your goal is to be aware of what's happening in your body, not to achieve an unrealistic level of discipline or dessert deprivation. I want you to become a nutrition detective, not a health nut. I want you to use food *for* yourself, not against yourself. The goal is not to be as thin as a model, or run a marathon, the goal is balance and awareness. As you create your own balanced relationship with food, you'll be amazed at how it spills over into the rest of your life. Not only will your energy and mental clarity increase, but you'll increase your ability to achieve goals in all areas of your life!

CHAPTER 1

Your Basics
for Optimal Health

TEN CORE PRINCIPLES FOR HEALTHY LIVING

EVERY DAY I RECEIVE LETTERS AND EMAILS from my readers telling me how much their health and energy has improved since they began incorporating the Ten Core Principles into their daily lives. I hear from couch potatoes whose beer bellies are shrinking; women who are walking a few miles every day and loving their newfound energy and muscle tone, senior citizens who have been able to stop taking their heart drugs, diabetics whose blood sugar is under control, and many more positive stories. The health benefits that you can derive from following these principles grow steadily as time passes.

The Ten Core Principles for Healthier Living is a guide for taking excellent care of yourself and embracing a healthy lifestyle. It's as simple as following these ten guidelines, which have evolved from more than thirty years of research, lecturing, and writing. Whether you implement only one or two of them or make a lifestyle overhaul, these ten principles work together or separately to improve your health. I'll be covering many of them in more detail as the book goes on. When you achieve optimal health, your energy level soars, which will help you keep your weight in check!

1. EAT WHOLE FOODS INSTEAD OF PROCESSED FOODS

Chronic diseases such as heart disease, diabetes, cancer, arthritis, osteoporosis, allergies, asthma, and autoimmune disorders are affecting more people in modernized nations than ever before. The medical research community has put much effort into pinpointing the causes of these diseases. They've come up with a wide variety of possible causes: genetic predisposition, too much fat in the diet, certain kinds of fat in the diet, certain chemicals in the environment, viruses, too much sugar, not enough calcium, and countless others. If you're trying to prevent or heal chronic disease, the mountain of conflicting advice based on the latest theories can be baffling.

I believe one of the most important answers to these questions is a simple one: A diet of refined, processed foods, rather than fresh, whole foods, is behind this increase in chronic diseases. The list of refined and processed foods includes canned and frozen food, refined white flour products (breads, bagels, baked goods, pasta, chips), sweets, meats such as bologna and hot dogs and countless other grocery store offerings that are long on sugar, salt, and fat and short on nutrition.

Processing foods strips them of their nutritional value. Refined foods tend to have strong, even addictive tastes compared to vegetables, fruits, and whole grains, but they are appetizing only because of the sugar, salt, oils, and other additives and flavorings they contain. Food manufacturers may add small amounts of vitamins and minerals to these products, but it hardly makes them equal in nutritional value to whole foods.

Whole foods are those that have undergone minimal or no processing and that are as close as possible to their natural state. The staples of a whole-food diet are fresh vegetables, whole grains, legumes (beans), fruit, raw nuts and seeds, and modest servings of organic meats, fish, poultry, and dairy products. Herbs, spice, and healthy oils add flavor and variety. (More diet specifics will be given later in the book.)

Contrary to popular belief, this kind of diet can be both delicious and satisfying. Your taste buds have grown accustomed to the powerful and addictive tastes of sugar, salt, and other artificial flavorings. Whole foods have more muted flavors that you need to adjust to if you've been eating primarily refined foods, but once you make the shift to whole foods, you'll feel so much better that you'll never want to go back.

A whole foods diet is one of the surest ways to keep your body youthful, energetic, slim, and free of disease. Of course, it's hard for some people to imagine eating nothing but whole foods. Even if you can't go all the way with it, try to replace processed foods with whole foods where you can. There are a few non-negotiables here, however.

Kick your sugar habit. Americans eat an average of approximately 155 pounds of sugar a year. Sugar—including white and brown varieties, fructose (fruit sugar), maple syrup, and honey—all cause blood sugar levels to fluctuate.

I'll explain this in greater detail later in the book, but in short, when you eat a sugary snack, your blood sugar rises way above normal. High blood sugar is harmful to the body in many ways, and so the pancreas comes to the rescue, pumping out plenty of insulin. Insulin's job is to pull sugar out of the blood and store it in the cells. It does its job so well that blood sugar levels plummet. You then suffer from the shakes, foggy thinking, and fatigue, and soon you're craving another dose of refined sugar.

Sugar depletes your body of B vitamins and the minerals magnesium and chromium. Deficiencies of these nutrients play a role in causing PMS. (In fact, research has shown that women who eat more sugar are more likely to have PMS.) Sugar suppresses your immune system, damages your kidneys, worsens allergies, and raises blood fats (cholesterol and triglycerides). It's true that some forms of sugar are less harmful than others—honey and maple sugar are less refined, and so have a less intense effect—but they'll put you on the sugar-addiction treadmill just as the others do. Your best bet is to break your sugar habit, and to reserve sweets for occasional use only.

Bypass the bread and pass on the pasta. When the medical community began to recommend a low-fat diet for weight loss and prevention of disease, throngs of health-minded people took notice. Rather than eating more vegetables and fruits, which are naturally low in fat, many turned to processed, packaged "low-fat" snacks and staples: pasta, pretzels, bread, and sugary snacks. Consumers were bombarded with advertising messages implying that if a food was low in fat, it was healthy. What they weren't told was that flour—especially white flour—has virtually the same effect on the body as sugar does. When wheat is stripped of its husk and oils and made into flour, it's called a *refined carbohydrate* and it essentially becomes sugar. Refined carbohydrates have virtually no nutritional value and cause blood sugar to swing rapidly up and down. Making these foods your mainstay is only slightly healthier than living on sweets.

If you can't live without bread, find a variety made with whole grains. It should say "whole grain" on the label, not just "whole wheat." For some people, corn tortillas are a more healthful alternative to bread. Use whole grains—brown rice, quinoa, barley, polenta, and millet—instead of pasta. They cook up quickly and taste great with vegetables. I'll talk about this in more detail too.

Use healthy oils. Recent research has revealed that the *amount* of fat you eat is less important than the *type* of fat you eat. There are three major categories of fats that exist in whole foods: saturated (found in meats, dairy products, palm kernel oil, and coconut oil), monounsaturated (found in olive, canola, and avocado oils), and polyunsaturated (found in other vegetable oils, nut and seed oils, and in soybean oil).

The saturation of a fat molecule describes the stability of that fat—its resistance to spoiling, or *oxidizing*. We're all familiar with the stale smell of rancid oils and fats. Oxidation of fats is a natural process that occurs when they are exposed to oxygen, creating free radicals, which damage cells. The more saturated the fat, the more resistant it is to oxidation. Thus, butter, a saturated fat, can sit in the fridge for days and not spoil, while an unsaturated oil such as corn or flax oil starts to go rancid the minute you open the bottle.

Antioxidants, such as vitamin C and vitamin E neutralize free radicals. If our free radical load is high and our antioxidant intake low, the overflow of oxidation can be highly destructive to our tissues. Excess free radicals are considered a common denominator in the causes of many chronic diseases, including heart disease, cancer and arthritis.

Saturated fats have been blamed for everything from heart disease to cancer, but they are only dangerous in excess. A small amount of butter or whole milk adds a lot of flavor and "mouth feel" to foods, and if you add these fats to your diet in moderate amounts they won't cause you any harm.

Polyunsaturated fats, such as corn oil, safflower oil, and cottonseed oil are very unstable and oxidize easily. Heating them to high temperatures for cooking produces many free radicals. The creation of partially hydrogenated oils is the food industry's attempt to solve this problem. By bombarding unsaturated oils with hydrogen atoms, food manufacturers create "hydrogenated oils" or "trans-fatty acids" that are more stable and resistant to spoilage. Although these fake fats were promoted for years as healthy (margarine is a prime example), we now know that they increase the risk of artery-clogging plaques and heart attacks. This increased risk is so well established that the FDA has decided that food manufacturers must include trans-fatty acid content on their labels. Hydrogenated fats are much worse for you than any saturated fat, and not much better than rancid unsaturated oils. I recommend avoiding all fake fats.

The gold standard of healthy oils is monounsaturated oil. Olive oil is your best bet; it's delicious, and the extra virgin varieties are only minimally processed. Canola oil, which is heavily processed to remove toxins, is best for baking and cooking foods that don't taste right with olive oil. These oils are only slightly less stable than saturated fats. The olive oil-rich Mediterranean diet has been shown to reduce the risk of heart disease.

Eat your fish. Deep-water fish such as salmon, mackerel, sardines, and cod are loaded with heart-healthy omega-3 fats. These fats are polyunsaturated, but in their natural form they do not go rancid before the fish goes bad, and they have potent anti-inflammatory effects, can lower cholesterol, protect against certain forms of cancer, and help to thin the blood (which helps prevent blood clots that cause heart attacks and strokes). Enjoy baked or poached fish at least twice a week.

Make raw foods a part of your daily diet. Raw foods contain enzymes that aid digestion and absorption of nutrients. Most people eat virtually no raw food. Cooking shuts off all enzyme activity and destroys water soluble vitamins such as vitamin C. Fresh fruit at breakfast or a green salad with dinner is an excellent way to add raw foods to your diet. Buy locally grown produce whenever you can; when it sits for long periods in trucks and on supermarket shelves, levels of enzymes and vitamins decrease.

2. DRINK PLENTY OF CLEAN WATER EVERY DAY

Your body is two-thirds water. Think of that water as a crystal-clear mountain lake. Now imagine that lake becoming stagnant because the streams that bring water into and out of it stop flowing. A stagnant lake becomes clouded and overgrown with algae. Now, imagine a campground being built next to the lake, bringing with it trash and sewage. More and more toxins come in, but with no moving fresh water to flush them away, the lake eventually becomes uninhabitable for the life forms that once thrived there.

This is what happens to your body when you consume the typical Western diet of processed foods, and don't drink enough water. If you don't constantly flush toxins from the water that makes up much of your body, they build up and can cause chronic disease. Even if you eat a whole-foods diet, you're still exposed to environmental toxins.

Drinking six to eight, eight-ounce glasses of pure water a day—not coffee, not juice, not milk, but water—is one of the simplest things you can do to improve your health. These results will be apparent within a few days: Your skin will glow, your bowels will move more regularly, and it will be easier for you to control your weight. In many cases, blood cholesterol levels drop. If you down your first glass or two when you get up in the morning, you'll find yourself becoming alert and awake without caffeine. If you keep a pitcher of water in your refrigerator, you'll always have a cool delicious beverage handy when you want it.

Please note that tap water simply isn't safe to drink. Depending on where you live and where your water comes from, the types of toxins that flow from your tap will vary. Heavy metals, benzene, chlorine, and carcinogenic agricultural chemicals are typical findings in tap water. Bottled water is expensive, and its quality isn't always assured. Anyone serious about improving their health should buy a water filtration system. You can buy them for a single tap or for your whole house.

3. GO ORGANIC

When you sit down to a meal, you don't intend to eat polychlorinated biphenlys, phthalates, bovine growth hormones, altered fruit and vegetable genes, organochlorine pesticides, antibiotics, or insecticides. If you aren't eating organic produce, grains, meats, eggs, and dairy products, it's a safe bet these toxins are a part of your daily diet. If you're eating processed foods, you're probably swallowing monosodium glutamate (MSG), aspartame, tartrazine, sodium benzoate, sodium nitrite, and a host of other additives and preservatives with your meals.

The chemicals listed above have been linked with a wide variety of chronic diseases, including cancer, liver disease, brain disease, autoimmune diseases, and diseases of the reproductive tract. Despite the food and chemical industries' efforts to minimize public knowledge of the harm brought on by these toxic substances, more and more people are taking the initiative to find out the truth—and they're buying organic.

Most livestock and poultry in North America are raised in crowded conditions and fed a diet that is far from optimal. As a result, these animals are riddled with diseases for which they are constantly fed antibiotics and other drugs. Before they are sent to market they are fed estrogens to fatten them up. Those drugs end up in your body when you eat their meat or eggs, or drink their milk. Vegetables, fruits, and grains that are not organic are sprayed with pesticides, fungicides, chemical fertilizers, weed-killers, and petrochemical-containing waxes.

The companies that make these chemicals insist that they are safe in the amounts people are exposed to. Sound familiar? They said that about

DDT, asbestos, and atrazine, too—chemicals that were finally banned when the evidence became overwhelming that they were damaging to all living creatures. When a new chemical is introduced, it goes through basic animal testing to be sure it doesn't cause birth defects or cancer. What I know now, however, is that often the harmful effects of chemical toxins don't appear until years after exposure; they can accumulate in the tissues of the body, and they can affect the offspring of people or animals who have been exposed in utero. Until there is overwhelming evidence of an approved chemical's toxicity, it remains on the market.

Mounting evidence shows that chemical toxins used on crops are harming humans, animals, and the environment. The interactions between different chemicals are impossible to predict, and the average person is exposed to dozens a day, in various combinations. Your best bet is to avoid chemicals whenever you can. Eating organic food is one way to accomplish this.

Organic foods are raised and grown under strict guidelines. Only natural methods are used on crops to get rid of pests and to encourage plants to grow. Animals raised organically are kept in more humane conditions and eat only organic feed. Organic products are more expensive, because the process of raising and growing them is more labor-intensive, but they're definitely worth it. The money spent on organics has made conventional farmers take notice. They recently tried to persuade the government to loosen the guidelines for what constitutes "organic." Rather than changing their mode of operations, the industry attempted to change the rules so that their present chemical-intensive practices could be considered organic! Fortunately, well-informed consumers made such an uproar about these proposed changes that they didn't go into effect.

If you only switch one part of your diet to organic, make it animal food—meat, poultry, dairy, and eggs. Some of the most dangerous toxins become concentrated in the fat of animal foods, and that's where you get the highest doses of these chemicals. One exception to this rule is fish, for which a set of organic labeling requirements hasn't been made. Eat more deep-water varieties such as salmon, cod, sardines, and mackerel. Tuna and swordfish have a higher level of mercury than most fish, so avoid eating them more than once a week. Generally shun bottom-dwelling seafood such as clams, oysters, lobster, and crabs, as they tend to be high in toxins that settle to the ocean floor.

Conventional cleaning supplies, bug spray, air fresheners, and beauty products also contain many potentially harmful ingredients. While it isn't necessary to find "organic" products for these purposes, substituting with natural alternatives (found in your health food store) will substantially lower your toxin load. You can also make your own cleaning supplies and insect repellents from natural ingredients. For example, most pests are repelled by aromatic oils such as rosemary, lavender and sage. White vinegar works for washing your windows! If you do a Web search for "natural pest control," you'll find plenty of detailed information. More nontoxic choices will become available commercially as people become more aware of the threat of exposure to these chemicals.

4. SUPPORT YOUR DIGESTIVE SYSTEM

If your digestive system isn't in good working condition, eating well and taking supplements won't help you much. A healthy stomach and small intestines work to break food down into proteins, carbohydrates, fats, vitamins, and minerals, and absorb them into the bloodstream. The small intestines also provide a highly selective barrier designed not to allow anything potentially toxic to pass into the circulation. A healthy large intestine maintains the proper balance of water and minerals in the body and provides a home for friendly bacteria, or probiotics. Probiotics make important vitamins and keep less friendly bacteria and yeasts, which occur naturally in the body, from becoming overgrown and causing illness.

Many of the chronic illnesses that are becoming so common—including irritable bowel syndrome, arthritis, asthma, allergies, chronic fatigue syndrome, depression, and autoimmune disease—can be traced back to imbalances in the digestive system. These imbalances are directly related to the consumption of the processed, nutrient-depleted Western diet. Conventional medicine has not yet recognized the importance of a balanced digestive system because of its "diagnose the symptom and prescribe a drug" mindset. Because the above diseases are often caused by a combination of conditions, including poor nutrition and digestion, conventional medicine has not had much success preventing or treating them.

Digestive problems can begin in the stomach, small intestines, or large intestines. These organs are interdependent, and as soon as one weakens, the others are compromised. A large proportion of people make insufficient stomach acid to break food down thoroughly. This is especially likely for people who suffer from heartburn or feelings of fullness for hours after eating.

You can support your digestive function with the right diet, but if you've been eating SAD (Standard American Diet) for some time, or if you have chronic indigestion or irritable bowel syndrome, you'll need a little extra help to get back on track. Try taking a digestive enzyme and betaine HCI (hydrochloric acid) supplement at each meal. Make sure the enzyme supplement contains protein, fat, and carbohydrate-digesting enzymes— protease, lipase, and amylase, respectively. To ensure that you have adequate friendly bacteria, keep a refrigerated probiotic supplement on hand, and take it between meals, especially if you have recently had to use antibiotics.

It's also important to get plenty of fiber in your diet, which you will do if you're eating the whole foods diet in Step 1. Fiber is found in unprocessed fruits and vegetables, whole grains, nuts, beans and seeds.

If you follow the diet guidelines and use these digestive supplements as needed, you'll get the very most out of your food.

5. VITAMIN AND MINERAL SUPPLEMENTS: THE BEST HEALTH INSURANCE

If you are committed to enjoying optimal health, be prepared to add nutritional supplements to your whole-foods diet. Vitamin and mineral supplements ensure that your body never lacks the nutrients it needs to perform all of its functions smoothly. A typical argument against supplements is that a healthy diet can supply all we need of these nutrients. This may be true of those who live in ideal conditions, with clean air and water, a diet composed only of whole, fresh organic foods grown in mineral-rich soil, and those who don't suffer from much stress. The rest of us must contend with foods that have been grown in depleted soil, and that have lost many of their nutrients from sitting on shelves and being cooked or processed. Pollution, toxic chemicals, and unprecedented levels of stress increase our need for certain nutrients. Nutritional supplements give us the extra support we need to stay healthy in an environment that is anything but healthful.

Research supporting the value of a high-quality multivitamin in the prevention of disease is piling so high that even its most vocal opponents are being forced to admit that it can't hurt and may even help. According to a study recently published in the *Western Journal of Medicine*, about 20 billion hospital health care dollars a year could be saved if all adults supplemented their diets with folic acid and vitamin E. Folic acid is important for prevention of neural tube defects and premature births, which cost hospitals millions of dollars a year. Vitamin E supplementation is one of the most important steps you can take to prevent heart disease, the number one killer in many Westernized countries, and the source of huge expenditures for high-tech surgeries and drugs. Extensive research has also shown the preventive value of supplementing with vitamin C, the B vitamins, carotenes, flavanoids, and minerals such as magnesium and calcium.

6. FIND A PHYSICIAN WHO IS OPEN TO ALTERNATIVE MEDICINE

Western medicine suffers from a crisis of faith. Tens of millions of people every year spend more money on alternative health choices than on conventional medicine. Those who seek health want to prevent disease, not just suppress symptoms with drugs and surgery when it's too late to heal.

As people become better informed about how their dietary choices and the use of supplements and preventive medicine affects their overall health, they are likely to find themselves in disagreement with their physicians (and insurance carriers) about the best way to treat an illness. Conventional physicians have been taught that tests, drugs, and surgeries are the best tools for practicing medicine. Many have had only rudimentary education about nutrition, and focus on diagnosing a disease and dispensing a prescription drug to treat it.

Many people complain that their physicians don't treat them as equals, that they are only interested in writing a prescription and getting them out of the office to make room for the next patient. This isn't necessarily the physician's fault; he or she is under enormous financial pressures and time constraints. Managed care is reinforcing the "diagnose and medicate" mindset in the medical professions. Many insurance carriers won't cover alternative treatments. Attaining optimal health may mean going against the grain, and perhaps paying out-of-pocket for alternative health services— at least until insurance carriers add these services to their plans. Some already offer coverage for nutritionally oriented acupuncture, or chiropractic treatments, but they are rare.

7. FIND NATURAL ALTERNATIVES TO PRESCRIPTION
AND OVER-THE-COUNTER DRUGS

A recent article in the *Journal of the American Medical Association* estimated that 140,000 Americans die each year from adverse drug effects (ADEs). This puts ADEs near the top of the list of leading causes of death in the U.S. Another study, this one from the FDA, stated that each year, approximately 938,000 people in the U.S. alone suffer "injuries" as a consequence of prescription drugs. Taxpayers and health insurance holders pay billions of dollars a year for the treatments and hospitalizations that result from these injuries. This doesn't take into account the subtle but significant changes in quality of life caused by side effects of prescription drugs.

Is Your Prescription Making You Gain Weight?

If you've recently put on pounds without changing your eating or exercise habits, a prescription or over-the-counter drug may be to blame. Dozens of drugs can change your metabolism, your mood or your appetite, resulting in weight gain. And it may be months before the change takes place. The biggest offenders include: hormone replacement drugs (e.g. the estrogens and progestins), antidepressant and antianxiety drugs (e.g. amitriptyline, clomipramine, alprazolam, phenelzine sulfate), cardiovascular and blood pressure-lowering drugs (e.g. guanethidine, betaxolol, pindolol, guanadrel, methyldopa), steroids (e.g. prednisone, beclovent, aerobid), and antihistamines (e.g. astemizole, loratadine).

Plenty of natural methods for combating depression and allergies and lowering blood pressure exist. Read our book, *Prescription Alternatives* for details!

In many instances, one drug's side effects are treated with another drug. I have dubbed this phenomenon the "drug treadmill." Many people who get on this treadmill end up feeling terrible, but would never think to attribute this to the effects of the drugs they use. Drug-related deaths and injuries are often the result of polypharmacy—the administration of several drugs to the same person at the same time. Mistakes in the dispensation of prescription drugs and drug interaction also contribute to the problem. Where do you think the real war on drugs needs to be waged?

Meanwhile, drug companies are getting richer and taking control of the health care systems. They sponsor continuing education for physicians, and publish biased studies about their latest wonder drugs. One of the most insidious tactics of the drug companies is their attempt to medicalize aging—establishing the notion that menopause is a disease to be treated with estrogen, that aging women should use powerful "designer estrogens" to prevent breast cancer, or that it's a matter of course to put aging people on blood pressure and cholesterol-lowering drugs. The considerable risks of these drugs are downplayed and their potential benefits trumpeted in slick TV ads and full-page, glossy advertisements in leading medical journals, magazines, and newspapers. Imagine the earning potential for the drug companies if the entire baby boomer population were to end up taking multiple medications from their fifties onward.

If you wish to avoid being caught up in this propaganda, adopt a three-pronged tactic. First, find a physician sympathetic to your wishes to stay off prescription and over-the-counter drugs. Second, if you already take any medications, talk to your physician about weaning yourself off of them as much as possible. When you go to your doctor, be prepared to ask about any alternative treatments you've read about. (If you are using medications, please don't discontinue them without your doctor's approval and help.) Third, if you absolutely must use a prescription drug, be as informed as possible about what it does in your body—its possible side effects, and any interactions it may have with other drugs or foods. Be sure you are given the lowest effective dose. Watch carefully for errors—know the generic and brand name of your prescription, and check every time you have it filled to be sure you're getting the right drug.

8. ADD MOVEMENT TO YOUR DAILY LIFE

For some people, exercise is a four-letter word. When you think of exercise, you might think of donning tight workout gear to slog away on a treadmill, or some other activity involving a great deal of sweat and strain. The latest research indicates, however, that mild to moderate exercise is as good for your health as intense exercise. On many levels, it's actually better for you to take a pleasant walk than to suffer through an exercise session that you hate. The most important thing is that this movement is something you enjoy; something you will do consistently for the rest of your life. The possibilities are endless—walking, running, swimming, dancing, bicycling, martial arts, aerobics classes, or any other mode of activity—and the choice is entirely yours.

This isn't to say that you shouldn't challenge yourself in your exercise program. For example, when you go for your walk, try to go at a brisk enough pace to bring out a light sweat and speed up your heartbeat. If you haven't exercised in some time, you may need to begin slowly and build up.

The simplest exercise is walking because all you need is a safe route and walking shoes with plenty of cushioning and support. Time spent covering a half-mile is certainly better for your body than time spent sitting on the couch, and walking one or two miles is better yet.

Aim to walk three to four miles, four to five times a week, but give yourself plenty of time to reach this goal, especially if you've been inactive. Once you're able to log three to four miles in an hour on a flat surface, try a hillier route. Keep challenging yourself, gradually, and your fitness level will improve and you'll keep your routine from becoming stagnant.

Three times weekly, use weights, rubber tubing, or your own body weight to strengthen your muscles, connective tissues, and bones. This is called resistance exercise. Stretch to keep joints supple. You can stretch after walking, and whenever else you think of it: as you sit in front of the television, read, or stand in line. Yoga, tai chi, and Qigong classes are terrific for staying limber and strong. You may also want to check into the many books and videotapes available to help you learn the proper form for strengthening and stretching exercises. Attending a few classes or hiring a trainer for one or two sessions should be enough to get you started.

You can also improve your fitness level simply by adding more movement to your everyday life. For example, park as far as possible from the store and walk. Ride your bicycle or walk rather than driving when you can. Take the stairs instead of the elevator. Rather than a chore, make housework and gardening an opportunity to bend, twist, reach, and squat. Remember: your body was made to move, and it works best when you move it regularly.

9. PAY ATTENTION

Next time you're about to pop a sugary snack into your mouth, stop for a moment. Are you really hungry, or just feeling in need of a little comfort food? Are you acting on force of habit, munching out of boredom? Or is it the time of day you always have a sweet snack? Perhaps you would gain just as much satisfaction from a tall glass of water, a piece of fruit, or a walk around the block. Take the time to listen to your body. If you listen for those subtle messages, your body will tell you what it needs.

The point here is to become aware of what you are doing. This doesn't mean you will decide against gobbling down that candy. You may well decide that despite it being bad for your body, you're going to eat it anyway. But then be attentive after you have eaten it, and notice the consequences of ingesting a concentrated dose of refined sugar.

This works in every area of your life. It isn't about punishing yourself for being "bad"—it's about simply noticing your habitual behaviors and the way those behaviors mold your life. If you remain attentive and aware of what you are doing and why, you'll find it easier to make healthy choices.

10. MANAGE STRESS WITH HEALTHY, LOVING RELATIONSHIPS, COMMUNITY, AND SPIRITUAL PRACTICE

An emerging science called psychoneuroimmunology is confirming what holistic, alternative medicine has known from the start: that our thoughts, feelings, attitudes, and relationships play a significant role in how well our bodies function. For example, when we are depressed, upset, or mourning, our immune system can be weakened, which makes us more vulnerable to disease.

To attain and maintain optimal health, it's best to cultivate healthy, open relationships with family and friends. Human beings need to feel as though they are an integral part of their community.

Joining local organizations, volunteering, and other meaningful work can help us to live longer and enjoy a better quality of life. Any meaningful relationship will see its share of interpersonal struggle, but we must be able to deal with the stress of conflict and work both within and in cooperation with others to find resolution. The best way to remain balanced in the midst of difficult situations is to make some kind of spiritual practice a regular part of your life.

It doesn't matter whether you choose to attend religious services, meditate, take tai chi or Qigong lessons, yoga classes, or engage in some other practice that links body, mind, and spirit. The important thing is that you quiet your mind, let go of your worries, and reestablish your center so that you know what is really true, what is right, what is important. Regular spiritual practice changes your whole outlook on life, and diminishes your unhealthy physical responses to stress. If a serious illness does catch up with you, a spiritual practice will give you the tools to cope with that stress and to marshal your body's own healing powers.

CHAPTER 2

Food Can Kill You or Heal You

YOU BECOME WHAT YOU EAT

Mary was in her late sixties and had developed arthritis. However, what mystified her was that it would flare up painfully for a few weeks, leaving her with a knobby knuckle on her hand or a stiff knee, and then disappear for months. For years, as her hands became more and more misshapen, she tried to figure out what caused her flare-ups. After reading my newsletter she discovered that certain foods can cause a flare-up of rheumatoid arthritis. She began to keep track of what she was eating and soon discovered that her worst flare-ups came in late summer when she was eating fresh tomatoes nearly every day. She stopped eating tomatoes, as well as potatoes and eggplants, which are in the same plant family (nightshade). Within a week her latest flare-up had calmed down, and she has had few of them since.

Like millions of older Americans, had she known that foods can cause arthritis, Mary could have avoided harmful anti-inflammatory drugs. Merely eliminating a few foods from her diet almost entirely solved her problem.

Greg, on the other hand, couldn't seem to give up jumbo hamburgers, and super-sized French fries. He figured he made up for this by having a low-fat cereal breakfast, but wasn't aware that he was eating the equivalent of 9 teaspoons of sugar in his serving of cereal. Although he was active enough to keep his weight down, he was developing prostate problems and was reluctant to take the drugs his doctor offered. However, he was waking several times a night to visit the bathroom and was having a hard time starting the flow of urine.

Greg went to one of my talks and found that the hormones in the hamburgers he was eating, combined with the deep-fried hydrogenated oils in the French fries and all the sugar in his cereal, were creating chronic inflammation in his prostate gland. He cut his burger intake down to once a week, cut out the fries, and started having whole grain toast with cashew butter for breakfast. Within a week his prostate problems diminished, and within a month, they had significantly improved. When he added a prostate supplement containing saw palmetto and zinc to his dietary changes, his symptoms were reduced to the point where they no longer bothered him.

One of the first steps in eating smart for optimal weight and health is to understand how profoundly what you eat can affect every part of your body. I'm not just talking about eating too much fat or sugar, I'm also referring to foods that can give some people arthritis, and others that can throw off your hormonal balance. Or how about foods that can shrink a prostate gland, and others that can unclog a heart? Doesn't it make sense that if we pick and choose the foods that will give us the best possible health we'll have the extra energy to go for a brisk walk before dinner? When you understand that your food is your medicine, you'll be more aware of how what you're eating affects everything from your mood and your blood pressure to your tendency to develop cancer or arthritis.

Folk medicine has told us for thousands of years that food is medicine. Some 2,500 years ago Hippocrates, a Greek who was the founder of medicine as we know it today, told his students, "Let thy food be thy medicine, and thy medicine be thy food." Conventional medicine seems to have forgotten this wisdom, but that doesn't mean you can't live by it.

About 60 trillion cells make up your body, each a complex mini-universe that experience billions of chemical reactions every minute of your life. What you eat is the fuel that gives them energy. Are you going to give your cells high-quality fuel for top performance? The choice is yours. Grasping the basics should inspire you to regularly notice how foods affect the working of your body.

Everybody is different, and what's good for one person may be poison to another. Remember Jack Sprat and his wife in the old nursery rhyme? One would eat no fat, and one would eat no lean. How do you respond to various foods? Do they give you a headache and gas, or do they make you feel energetic and clear-headed? Do you feel like you have a hangover the morning after you eat certain foods, or do you feel strong and well-nourished? Do your joints ache after you eat what you thought was a big, healthy salad? Does a glass of wine give you a headache? These physical indications are all feedback from your body about what's working and what's not. It's up to you to keep track of the information and tailor your diet to fit what's best for your body.

WHAT DID OUR ANCESTORS EAT?

Medical anthropologists look at how the human body works, and at how humans behave, and then go back through the ages to figure out why we evolved with those particular functions and behaviors.

For tens of thousands of years, our ancestors evolved without artificial light. They went to sleep when it got dark, and awoke with the sun. In response, the human brain learned to secrete the brain chemical melatonin in response to darkness, to help bring on sleep. Furthermore, in the summers, when longer days bring more light, humans had more food to eat, and put on more weight than in the winter, when days were shorter and daylight hours fewer. Accordingly, our bodies developed biochemical behaviors in response to longer or shorter days. Some medical anthropologists theorize that leaving the lights on into the wee hours, and sleeping in rooms that aren't completely dark, sends a signal to our brains that it's perpetual summer, and that we should be putting on weight. To maintain a healthy weight, they recommend going to bed early in a completely dark room, and getting up with the sun as much as possible.

Another aspect of anthropological medicine that is being examined in some detail involves what types of foods (and in what proportions) our ancestors ate. Another way of looking at it is, if humans evolved over 50,000 years eating a certain way, then we can be certain that our genes have evolved to create optimal health based on that way of eating. Those who ate in a way that enhanced their health and thus their survival got to pass their genes along more often than those who didn't.

The U.S. Department of Agriculture (USDA) has created their so-called food pyramid to tell us how we should eat in order to be healthy. I refer to it as "so-called" because its content is dictated more by food industry politics than by nutrition science. Their pyramid suggests that the bulk of our diet should be grains and cereals, but does not distinguish between refined carbohydrates and whole grains. It also does not differentiate what types of fats or proteins we should be eating. Current nutritional wisdom also preaches that calories are calories are calories, regardless of whether they come from fats, proteins or starches. Obviously those who believe this dogma have never studied human biochemistry, because the type of calories you eat makes all the difference in what happens inside your body.

Unfortunately, the construction of this pyramid is primarily influenced by those in power in the food industry, and the millions of Americans who have been struggling to follow it—under instructions from teachers, dieticians and physicians—are getting fatter and unhealthier by the decade.

So how do we figure out what's best for us to eat without bias from money and politics? Why not start by looking back at what our ancestors ate? After all, our Paleolithic hunter-gather ancestors of 50,000 years ago spent millennia evolving into what we are today. Agriculture, or the tending of crops, has only been around for about 10,000 years. Before that, our ancestors may have gathered what they could find along the way, but grains were not a primary staple of their diet the way they have been since we began tilling the soil and planting seeds. In fact, most grains are indigestible unless they are ground, and evidence of grinding stones didn't show up until about 15,000 years ago. According to Dr. Loren Cordain, a professor at Colorado State University in Fort Collins and an expert in the area of Paleolithic nutrition, wheat wasn't found in Europe until about 5,000 years ago. He estimates that rice showed up in Asia and corn showed up in Mexico and Central America about 7,000 years ago. Thus, the inclusion of grains in the diet is a fairly recent event in human evolutionary history, yet the USDA's message is that we should subsist on them.

Dr. Cordain states that when humans began farming they became shorter, infant mortality rates increased, life spans shortened, they were prone to more infections, iron deficiency anemia, cavities and weaker bones. What did we eat prior to agriculture? Mostly meat supplied by many different types of small and large animals. Our ancestors took advantage of every edible part of the kill, including such nutritionally rich parts as the liver and kidneys, the brain and the bone marrow, but favored the fattiest parts. In a collection of essays titled *Ice Age Hunters of the Rockies*, the authors tell us that our North American ancestors ate mammoth, camel, sloth, bison, mountain sheep, beaver, pronghorn antelope, elk, mule deer, horse, llama, and large members of the dog family. Bear and wild pig were eaten throughout the world. Our Paleolithic ancestors also ate a variety of eggs, as well as insects, fish, birds, and reptiles—all of which supplied high quality protein. This was supplemented by such foods as roots, leaves, bulbs, berries, nuts, seeds, and in the summer, fruit.

In light of this, it's no wonder that our health is poor. We subsist on a diet of mostly grains and refined sugars, when our bodies evolved eating meats, low-sugar vegetables, nuts, and seeds! Dr. Cordain believes when cereal grains provide 10 percent or more of our daily caloric intake, our health begins to seriously suffer. With this in mind, let's take a look at how food can be our medicine when we eat more like our ancestors did.

HAUNTED BY HEART DISEASE

Most American men are haunted by the threat of heart disease. They tend to die younger than women, and they die of heart attacks in greater numbers than women do. If more men realized how easily they can keep their hearts happily beating into their older years, we could cut deaths from heart attacks in men by 20 percent within a few years. However, heart attacks are also the leading cause of death among women, so let's not fool ourselves into thinking this is just a guy problem: It's just that the women seem to get a few more years of life before they have their heart attack.

A heart attack is the final result of a condition that has usually been building for years inside the arteries of the heart. Heart disease is a chronic or ongoing disease. You can't see or feel plaque sticking to your arteries: It's a silent process. As the arteries are damaged over the years, the hard, sticky plaque deposits are laid down by the body in an attempt to patch things up, but eventually they narrow the blood vessels. The common name for this phenomenon is hardening of the arteries; your doctor calls it arteriosclerosis.

By now, we're all aware that nutrition plays a major role in both prevention and treatment of heart disease. Even if you once ate recklessly, and even if you've had a heart attack, changing your diet may prevent future cardiac arrest, and even halt or reverse arterial damage, and help restore arteries to health. Your body has a remarkable ability to heal itself, even as you age, and food is its best medicine.

WHAT ABOUT CHOLESTEROL?

There is no one single cause of heart disease, but there are plenty of known risk factors. Besides age, gender, and other conditions that may be out of our control, we *can* control our smoking, weight, and diet. We can learn how to manage stress better, and protect ourselves when we're around known toxins such as pesticides and solvents.

Although high blood pressure and high cholesterol are not direct causes of heart disease as conventional medicine would have you believe, they are symptoms of heart disease, and the steps you take to reduce these symptoms can help heal your heart disease. Just keep in mind that if the prescription drugs that lower blood pressure and cholesterol really worked to "cure" heart disease, the number of people dying from heart disease each year would have dropped dramatically in the past few decades, as millions of Americans have been put on these drugs. But that is definitely not what's happening. Drugs are not the answer.

Top Ten Cholesterol-Busting Foods

Apples

Berries

especially blueberries and raspberries

Carrots

Fish

especially salmon, mackerel, herring, sardines, cod, tuna, trout

Grapefruit

Legumes

(a.k.a. beans)

Prunes

Soy products

such as miso and tofu

Whole grains

including rice, barley, millet, oats, wheat, and rye

Yogurt

You've probably heard that a useful measure of risk for heart disease is the ratio of your "good" cholesterol (HDL—high-density lipoprotein) to the "bad" cholesterol (LDL—low-density lipoprotein). However, what's really harmful is oxidized, or rancid LDL cholesterol, which contributes to damaging your arteries. HDL cholesterol, on the other hand, protects your arteries from LDL. Therefore, you want your levels of HDL cholesterol to be high. You don't hear much about HDL cholesterol from conventional medicine, because cholesterol-lowering drugs don't do a very good job of raising HDL levels.

Contrary to popular opinion, eating high-cholesterol foods such as eggs and red meat does *not* give you high cholesterol levels. Your body makes most of your good and bad cholesterol out of the sugars and starches that you eat, and gets a small percentage from cholesterol in the diet. Excess cholesterol is simply excreted from the body. If you eat highly fatty red meat three times a day, your body might start to have a hard time excreting the cholesterol from your blood, but if your fat intake is moderate, high cholesterol foods won't hurt you. In fact, too little cholesterol is bad for you. All of your steroid hormones (progesterone, estrogen, testosterone, DHEA, cortisol) are made from cholesterol, and it plays an important role in brain function. Research has even shown that people whose cholesterol is too low can become depressed and more prone to suicide.

But why do so many people have excessively high cholesterol levels? It's mostly from eating too many trans-fatty acids (such as partially hydrogenated vegetable oils) and too much sugar, which creates chronic inflammation in the body and raises cholesterol levels.

BAN THE TRANS FATTY ACIDS

Want to know what's playing a big role in destroying the arteries of millions of Americans? It's trans-fatty acids (partially hydrogenated oils), which are found in almost all processed foods—margarine, cookies, chips, breads, canned sauces, puddings, condiments, and frozen foods. The hot grease that French fries are cooked in may be at the top of the trans-fatty acids danger list.

These fats are rarely found in nature, and your body does not know how to process them properly. Partially hydrogenated oils were originally created because unsaturated oils such a corn and safflower oil are extremely unstable and easily go rancid, which also creates a known risk for heart disease. When vegetables oils are partially hydrogenated they can sit on supermarket shelves for months and not go bad: good for manufacturers, but bad for your blood vessels! Therefore, one key to a healthy heart is to avoid processed foods as much as possible, and especially those that contain partially hydrogenated oils.

You may be surprised to learn that certain whole foods can actually save arteries and prevent heart disease. These foods include: seafood, fruits, vegetables, nuts, oat bran, legumes, onions, garlic, olive oil, and foods high in vitamins C, E, and beta carotene. It should come as no surprise to you that eating fewer trans-fatty acids and more of these healthy heart foods will also help you lose weight!

EAT MORE FISH FOR A HEALTHY HEART AND WEIGHT LOSS

The omera-3 fatty acids found in fish are some of your most effective weapons against heart disease. A study of 6,000 middle-aged American men showed that those who ate the equivalent of marine fat in a one-ounce bite of mackerel or three ounces of bass a day were 36 percent less likely to die of heart disease than those who ate less or none at all. By eating a five-ounce serving of oily fish like salmon, mackerel, or sardines at least twice a week, your odds of a heart attack are a third less than if you simply followed a low-fat, high-fiber diet with no fish.

Here are some of the beneficial effects that eating fish has on your heart: it keeps blood slippery and smooth and less likely to clot; lowers triglycerides, a type of fat that increases the risk of heart disease; helps keep blood vessels open; lowers blood pressure; is beneficial for the brain; reduces your need for insulin; and keeps cholesterol balance healthy.

If you don't like fish, you can find fish oil capsules at your health food store, but be sure they're well preserved and purified; rancid or toxic fish oil will do you more harm than good!

BRING ON THE OLIVE OIL, AVOCADOS, AND NUTS

You've probably been taught to avoid olive oil, avocados, and nuts because they're high calorie, high-fat foods. This is nutritional nonsense. These are nutritionally dense foods that contain many health benefits packed into each ounce. The fat in olive oil is monounsaturated, which lowers LDL ("bad") cholesterol, while slightly raising HDL ("good") cholesterol. It also has an antioxidant quality that protects arteries against the oxidative damage that can make cholesterol dangerous. Monounsaturated fat, which can also be found in almonds, hazelnuts, walnuts, and avocados, is heart-protective. Researchers found that test subjects who went on a low-fat diet that shunned nuts reduced their cholesterol by an average of 6 percent, but when they added walnuts to their diet, their cholesterol decreased by another 13 percent. The key is to eat a handful of nuts a day as part of a healthy snack. Nuts are also loaded with vitamins and minerals, so they're a great nutritional package.

Australian researchers discovered that avocado eaters (½ to 1½ avocados per day) improved their cholesterol twice as much as non-avocado-eating low-fat dieters.

Foods for the Heathy Heart

- Consume at least 30 grams of fiber daily.

- Eliminate trans-fatty acids (hydrogenated oils) from your diet.

- Eat plenty of garlic and onions.

- Eat red meat in moderation.

- Eat more fish (salmon, mackerel, cod, halibut, bass, albacore tuna, sardines, herring).

- Eat more nuts. (Raw or dry roasted, lightly salted or unsalted—but avoid nuts that have been roasted in peanut oil!)

- Eat plenty of fresh, organic fruits and vegetables.

- Eat more soy foods such as miso, tempeh, and tofu.

- Use olive oil and small amounts of butter when you need fat or oil in your food.

THEY STINK, BUT THEY'RE WORTH IT!

Onions, garlic, chives, leeks, and shallots are well-known food members of the *allium* family of plants. Although there are more than 500 members of the *allium* family, these five are the best known.

People who eat garlic on a daily basis tend to be healthy folks; this lifestyle habit can reduce the risk of death from heart attack by as much as 66 percent after three years, and can reduce high blood pressure and blood cholesterol by 10 percent. Researchers believe that a steady infusion of garlic can wash away some arterial plaque and help prevent future damage, probably because of a conglomeration of some 15 different antioxidants that neutralize artery-destroying agents. Garlic also reduces joint pain, body aches, and asthma, and improves vigor, energy, libido, and appetite. Now we all know that if our hearts are pumping well, we're breathing well, and our joints don't ache, we'll be more willing to exercise when we wake up in the morning.

Onions are close cousins of garlic that have many of the same health benefits and bring delicious flavor to everything from eggs and eggplant to soups and salads. Onions are among our most ancient foods, and are so popular in all cultures today that they rank sixth among the world's top vegetable crops.

I'm sure you're familiar with the red, white, and yellow onions found in the supermarket. And of course, most of us have had pearl onions or the slightly larger boiling onions in some form at holiday meals mixed with peas or covered with a cream sauce. Shallots, which are like a combination of onion and garlic, are widely used in Europe. Scallions are simply the green tops of immature onions. They have a mild flavor and are particularly delicious floating on the top of miso soup. Chives are close relatives of onions that look like scallions but are more delicate and grass-like. They are most often used to season salads or as a visually pleasing garnish.

All of these alliums except chives are bulbs with a similarly strong odor that becomes stronger when they are cut or bruised. Onions in particular are known for making us cry as we prepare them. Slicing into an onion creates a chemical reaction between enzymes and sulfur-containing amino acids that releases sulfuric acid, causing eye irritation. The older the onion, the harder you'll cry! Cooking neutralizes these strong substances and turns onions sweet. In fact, some components of onions are fifty times sweeter than white sugar.

Onions contain more than 100 sulfur-containing compounds, some thought to inhibit the growth of cancer and most specifically to prevent stomach and colon cancer. In Chinese medicine, these compounds are believed to be responsible for the onion's ability to detoxify the body, including removing heavy metals and parasites; and for improving the absorption and utilization of protein. They can also deactivate excess estrogen, inhibit carcinogens and enzymes that cause cancer, reduce blood pressure, raise good cholesterol (HDL), and prevent the formation of blood clots.

As if all that wasn't enough, onions are also very potent antioxidants. Red and yellow onions and shallots are the richest dietary source of quercetin, a potent antioxidant bioflavonoid. These antioxidants are sure to play a part in onion's power to ward off colds, allergies, asthma, and bronchitis, as well as other inflammatory reactions, bacteria, and viruses.

Onions are also a good source of the mineral selenium, which has been shown in studies to be protective against prostate and colon cancer. Selenium may enable the onion to cleanse the body, especially of heavy metals, by binding with them to form compounds that are then flushed out of the system. Selenium also acts as an antioxidant which specifically has the ability to neutralize rancid fats which might otherwise cause damaging oxidative reactions. Studies show that geographical areas with the higher amounts of selenium in the soil have lower rates of cancer and stroke. Other studies show that populations with the highest blood selenium have the lowest cancer rates.

The down side of the onion family can be heartburn, gas and, and of course, the dreaded onion breath. If you're experiencing heartburn and gas when you eat onions you may be sensitive to the sulfur compounds contained in the *allium* family plants. These compounds can even cause a skin rash and asthma in some sensitive people. In that case, I recommend you eliminate them from your diet.

As for onion breath, you have a number of choices. You can feed your friends and family members lots of onions, so nobody will notice. Or you can chew on a sprig of parsley after a meal with onions.

Onions are one of those foods that should be a staple in everyone's diet (as long as you're not sensitive to them). You can't beat the health benefits, and the flavor can turn even the most boring dish into a gourmet meal.

BEANS MAKE YOU SLIM AND HEALTHY

Dried beans or legumes are one of nature's least-expensive, fastest acting, and safest healthy-heart foods. They contain at least six cholesterol-cutting weapons, they lower blood pressure, and their fiber prevents colon cancer. A cup of beans—soy, black, navy, lentil, pintos, kidneys, or chickpeas—a day can cut LDL cholesterol by 20 percent after about three weeks. I'll go into more detail about eating beans later in the book.

FIBER IS GOOD FOOD

Any type of fiber, eaten at least with every meal, will help reduce heart disease risk. And you don't need to choke down those gummy psyllium powders (e.g. Metmucil) to get it. Fiber is the non-digestible part of fruits, vegetables, grains, nuts and seeds that passes all the way through the digestive system. Although it's not a nutrient, it has many beneficial effects on the digestive system, as it helps absorb toxins, moves waste out of the bowels, and prevents constipation. The medicinal effects of fiber have been known for thousands of years, but only in recent years have scientists begun to understand its importance in the daily diet as a means of preventing disease and maintaining health.

Here are some good sources of fiber to choose from that also give you lots of nutrition in each serving. Each listing contains between 2 and 3 grams of fiber.

> **Apples** (2 medium)
> **Apricots** (4 raw)
> **Artichoke** (½)
> **Avocado**, California (1)
> **Bananas** (1½ raw)
> **Beans**, kidney, pinto (⅓ cup, cooked)
> **Beans**, lima (¼ cup, cooked)
> **Beans**, white (½ cup, cooked)
> **Cantaloupe** (¼)
> **Cauliflower** (¾ cup, raw)
> **Cereals** (whole grain, ¾ cup to 1 cup)
> **Chickpeas** (½ cup, cooked)
> **Corn** (½ cup)
> **Eggplant** (1 cup, cooked)
> **Figs** (2 medium)
> **Grapefruit**, white (½)
> **Greens**, collard, kale, mustard, turnip (1 cup, cooked)
> **Lettuce**, dark green or loose-leaf (1 cup)
> **Oat bran** (⅓ cup, dry)
> **Oatmeal** (¾ cup, cooked)
> **Okra** (¾ cup)
> **Potato** (¾ medium, baked)
> **Strawberries** (1 cup)
> **Squash**, zucchini, summer (¾ cup)
> **Prunes** (5)
> **Whole grain bread** (1 slice)

VEGGIES ARE HEART HELPERS

If there's one thing that all nutritional experts agree on, it's that fresh vegetables are just about the healthiest food you can eat, and are also the food most lacking in the typical Western diet. If you fill up on salads, or stir-fried veggies, or broccoli, you're more likely to be nutritionally satisfied and less likely to binge on junk food.

Fresh vegetables contains loads of valuable nutrients, few calories, plenty of fiber, enzymes to help you digest, and a potpourri of phytonutrients, most of which we don't even have names for yet. Some of our favorite healthy veggies are broccoli, cauliflower, bok choy, romaine lettuce, carrots, green beans, yellow squash, fresh corn on the cob (technically a grain), red peppers and cucumbers.

TAKE A DEEP BREATH, RELAX, AND EAT
TO LOWER YOUR BLOOD PRESSURE

Although obesity and stress are undoubtedly the biggest causes of high blood pressure, food can make a big difference in relaxing your blood vessels. Once again, fish is near the top of the list for natural blood pressure remedies. Regularly eating fatty fish such as cod, mackerel, and salmon lowers blood pressure.

If your minerals are out of balance, it can push the fluid levels in your cells out of balance, and that can raise blood pressure. This is particularly true of deficiencies of the minerals magnesium and potassium. Magnesium-rich foods include nuts and leafy green vegetables. Potassium-rich foods include bananas, white potatoes, yogurt, dried apricots, cantaloupes, and orange juice.

Garlic and cruciferous vegetables such as broccoli, cabbage, and kale contain sulfide compounds that can also help lower blood pressure.

DR. MINDELL'S NATURAL BLOOD PRESSURE LOWERING PROGRAM

1. One of the best—and simplest—ways to reduce blood pressure is to drink plenty of clean water. Depending on your body size, you should be drinking 6 to 10 glasses of water per day. Try it!

2. Exercise moderately at least 20 minutes every day or 45 minutes three to four times a week.

3. Eat a diet emphasizing whole, fresh foods, especially vegetables, grains, and plenty of fiber. Avoid refined, packaged and processed foods, and sweets.

4. Limit alcohol consumption to 2 drinks per day or less.

5. Stop smoking.

Daily Vitamins for Lowering Blood Pressure

(The specific forms of the vitamins are given because they are best absorbed and assimilated.)

- **Vitamin C**: 1,000 to 2,000 mg daily, in an esterfied C complex form
- **Vitamin E**: 400 to 500 IU daily as mixed tocopherols
- **Magnesium**: 500 to 1000 mg in the aspartate or glycinate form
- **Calcium**: 500 to 600 mg daily in a glycinate or hydroxy apatite form
- **Zinc**: 5 to 10 mg per day

Herbs for Lowering Blood Pressure

(Follow instructions on the bottle for the optimal dosage.)

Cayenne	**Dandelion**
Dong Quai	**Garlic**
Gingko biloba	**Ginseng**
Hawthorn	**Reishi mushrooms**

Foods For Lowering Blood Pressure

Fresh fruits and vegetables
Fresh celery (4 stalks a day has been known to significantly reduce blood pressure)
Cold water, deep sea fish (cod, mackerel, sardines, salmon, herring)
Olive oil (instead of vegetable oils or butter)

ARTHRITIS AND FOOD: THE LEAKY GUT CONNECTION

When it comes to arthritis, and especially rheumatoid arthritis, your favorite food could be your worst enemy. Specific compounds in food, including fat, can regulate the functioning of hormone-like biochemicals called prostaglandins that help control inflammation, pain, and other arthritic symptoms. In addition, some folks can be sensitive to specific foods, and we'll explain why shortly. So, on the one hand, you might eat certain foods that, in fact, act as drugs to relieve the pain, swelling, fatigue, and stiffness of arthritis. On the other hand, avoiding one or more foods may cure you quickly and permanently.

The sensitivities that some people have to certain foods which then cause arthritis symptoms are often called food allergies, but they're not allergies in the traditional sense—they do not cause a rash or hives, or cause the throat to swell. One doctor suggests that 60 to 80 percent of arthritis sufferers could benefit from dietary changes, and one double-blind test concluded that as many as 85 to 90 percent of patients have food-triggered arthritis.

The biggest culprits in causing arthritis symptoms are from the nightshade family of plants—tomatoes, potatoes, eggplants, and peppers. Other common offenders include citrus, corn, wheat, and dairy products. If you have arthritis, it's well worth it to try what's called an elimination diet.

To do an elimination diet, for one week keep a list of every type of food that you eat, from meals to snacks to drinks. Then go back and circle the foods that appear on your list every day. Think about which of these foods that you feel you can't do without for a day: that's the one to eliminate. Don't worry, you probably won't need to give it up forever. You may be surprised to learn that the food you most crave is the one causing your joints to ache. That's because when we're sensitive to foods, it can cause the body to release adrenaline-like substances in defense, which perks up our energy for a little while. We crave those foods because we want that temporary energy boost.

How do these foods cause arthritis? The most likely theory is that they cause irritation to the lining of the intestines, which allows miscroscopic particles of the food to escape into the bloodstream, which is why this collection of symptoms is known as leaky gut syndrome. Because they haven't been properly tagged by the immune system, these food particles are perceived as invaders and are attacked. This attack process can cause inflammation in many parts of the body, including the joints.

But let's get back to the elimination diet. For example, maybe it's potatoes that you can't live without every day—then you would want to eliminate all nightshade foods from your diet for at least three weeks. If your symptoms improve or even get better, avoid nightshade foods for at least three months. (If symptoms don't improve, pick another food to eliminate. If you decide to eliminate a very common food such as wheat or dairy products, you'll have to read labels very carefully to avoid them.) After three months, eat a moderate amount of potato first thing in the morning. Notice any symptoms that show up during the next few days, such as digestive problems, a stuffy nose or headache. If you do have symptoms, eliminate that food completely for at least three months. After that don't eat it more than once or twice a week.

Depending on your ethnic heritage (Northern European, Asian, Mediterranean, African, etc.), you may be more prone to certain food sensitivities than others. For example, while many Northern Europeans can tolerate dairy products as adults, Asians and Native Americans are almost always intolerant to cow's milk. Listed below are the top twenty foods that typically provoke rheumatoid arthritis symptoms in Northern Europeans, from the worst culprits, to the least. Corn and wheat are by far the worst offenders:

Corn	Milk	Beef	Grapefruit	Butter
Wheat	Oats	Coffee	Tomato	Lamb
Bacon/Pork	Rye	Malt	Peanuts	Lemon
Oranges	Eggs	Cheese	Sugar (cane)	Soy

ANOTHER FOOD REMEDY FOR ARTHRITIS

One of the newest yet oldest cures for arthritis symptoms is ginger. This spicy root has been used for centuries in Asian medicine to treat achy joints, and now Western researchers are finding that ginger's pain-banishing properties have some real science behind them. You can find a variety of ginger extracts at your health food store—follow dosage directions on the container. You can also incorporate ginger into your cooking and make it into a tea.

AVOID NSAIDs IF POSSIBLE

Non-steroidal anti-inflammtory drugs (NSAIDs) such as aspirin and ibuprofen can block the formation of prostaglandins that induce swelling, but they can have major side effects, including stomach ulcers. In fact, some NSAIDs can eat through the stomach lining and get into the bloodstream where they promote the development of food sensitivities.

BANISH THAT POUNDING HEADACHE
BY WATCHING WHAT YOU EAT

Headaches come in many different forms, from dull and throbbing, to sharp and stabbing, to debilitating migraines. Headaches are triggered by numerous culprits, including muscle tension, caffeine, blood sugar imbalances, hangover, emotional stress, sinus congestion or infection, hormone imbalance, high blood pressure, eyestrain, fever, gum chewing and overexertion.

Often headaches are triggered by a sensitivity to certain chemicals such as the phenylalanine found in aspartame (e.g. Equal and NutraSweet), monosodium glutamate (MSG often found in Chinese food), or nitrates (preservatives found in hot dogs and lunch meats). Another potential source of headache is a substance called tyramine which is found in red wine, bananas, cheese, chicken, chocolate, citrus fruits, cold cuts, herrings, onions, peanut butter, pork, smoked fish, sour cream, vinegar, and fresh-baked yeast products. Any type of alcohol may cause trouble for someone who is prone to headaches. Experiment with eliminating these substances from your diet to see if your headaches improve.

Calcium and magnesium, effective in easing premenstrual and menopausal symptoms, can also be useful for preventing headaches. Women who get 200 mg of calcium daily have significantly fewer headaches than those who don't, and this amount is easily eaten in yogurt, tofu, and almonds. If you eat nuts, seeds and green veggies, and live in an area that has hard water on tap, you're probably getting enough magnesium. Those most at risk of magnesium deficiency are heavy drinkers (alcohol), people who use diuretics to lower blood pressure, and women on supplemental estrogen without progesterone to balance it.

Aspartame: No Substitute for Sugar

Aspartame, marketed under the brand names NutraSweet and Equal, among others, is found in more than 5,000 food and drink products and is used by more than half the adults in the United States—100 million-plus people. When it first came out, people with a sweet tooth and a weight problem thought they could finally have their cake and eat it too: Aspartame is 200 times sweeter than sugar, contains no calories, and doesn't have the bitter aftertaste of saccharin. Aspartame is virtually hidden in hundreds of products from chewing gum and laxatives to jello and yogurt, once again, a good reason to avoid processed foods and read labels closely when you do eat them!

As soon as it gets into the stomach, aspartame breaks down into its components, the amino acids, aspartic acid and phenylalanine, and a methyl ester which breaks down into methyl alcohol (also called wood alcohol), a known poison, which then breaks down into formaldehyde, a known neurotoxin.

You might think that because amino acids are natural substances, and there are only small amounts of methyl alcohol in a can of diet soda or a box of jello, that aspartame should be harmless. And for some people that very well may be true. But for many others it opens a Pandora's box of health problems ranging from annoying to lethal, particularly if they fall into the all-too-common pattern of downing many cans of diet soda every day.

The amino acid aspartic acid is an "excitotoxin," a substance essential to normal brain function. Part of its job description is to excite neurons, but in excess it excites them to death, and we certainly don't want to be killing off brain cells! For this reason, the nervous system maintains exquisite control of this substance, along with glutamate, another excitotoxin found in the flavor-enhancer MSG (monosodium glutamate). Aspartic acid and glutamate are even more dangerous when combined, making a diet soda and an MSG-containing meal a double whammy. This excitatory and dying process caused by an excess of excitotoxins results in "brain" symptoms such as headaches, dizziness, and memory loss, common among aspartame users who are sensitive to this substance.

Phenylalanine, another essential brain chemical, can also be dangerous. For years an excess has been known to cause brain damage, as well as aggressive and hyperactive behavior. One in 15,000 babies is born with an enzyme deficiency that causes excess phenylalanine, called phenylketonuria (PKU). If foods containing phenylalanine aren't eliminated from their diets early on, babies can become severely re- tarded as a result of the brain damage caused by the phenylalanine. As a result, the consequences of excessive phenylalanine have been well studied and documented. Those of us who don't have PKU can safely eliminate phenylalanine from the body, but it's just common sense to avoid drinking something that could create an excess. Excess phenylalanine may also contribute to obesity and has been linked to schizophrenia and seizures.

Probably the most common complaint about aspartame is head- aches, ranging from annoying to severe. Other common complaints include dizziness, memory loss, foggy thinking, irritability, anxiety, phobias, vision problems (blurring, bright flashes, tunnel vision), and depression. Other side effects are itchiness (which can also be caused by the enormous amounts of caffeine put in diet sodas), rashes, dry eyes, slurred speech, high blood pressure, tremors, abdominal pain, ringing in the ears, swelling of the throat, diarrhea, and, (I kid you not) weight gain.

Nearly everyone but the FDA agrees that aspartame can have a toxic effect on the fetal brain and should not be used by pregnant women. Since so many substances pass from mother's milk into an infant, it's also not advisable for nursing mothers to consume aspar- tame. I'm convinced that aspartame is the cause of much hyperac- tivity and learning disabilities in children, and I've noticed that many people who drink diet sodas have what I call the "excitotoxin twitch," jerky movements of the head, arms and hands. This could be caused by the aspartame, or by a combination of aspartame and caffeine. Some 78 percent of complaints about food and drugs reported to the FDA are about aspartame! Just think if an herbal medicine generated just one percent of the calls to the FDA. It would be yanked off the shelves faster than you can say "excitotoxin!"

Aspartame causes a drop in blood sugar that over time can cre- ate blood sugar imbalances and insulin resistance. Even though it is not sugar, the sweet taste on the tongue causes the body to release insulin.

Aspartame also causes menstrual irregularities, and the cause of this is not a mystery either. Excitotoxins play an important role in how the hypothalamus, a tiny gland in the brain, regulates hormones. Phe- nylalanine is a precursor to the brain chemicals norepinephrine and dopamine, both of which play important roles in regulating pituitary hormones, which in turn regulate such hormones as thyroid, growth hormone, prolactin and oxytocin. An imbalance of these important substances could have a profound effect on a growing child.

If you want more information about the effects of excitotoxins on the brain, I recommend the book, *Excitotoxins: The Taste that Kills*, by Russell Blaylock, M.D.

INDIGESTION

If you have gas, abdominal pain, rumbling noises in your stomach, a bloated feeling, nausea, vomiting, a burning sensation after eating, or you belch a lot, you may have a disorder in the stomach and intestines. These disorders could include intestinal obstruction, malabsorption, peptic ulcers, or problems with the pancreas, liver, or gallbladder. Or, more likely, you may just have plain old indigestion.

Indigestion can be caused by swallowing air when you chew or gulp food down. Drinking liquids with your meals can dilute the enzymes that aid digestion. Alcohol, vinegar, caffeine, and greasy or spicy foods can irritate the digestive tract. Food allergies, milk intolerance, or psychological stress can also cause it.

Food not digested properly can ferment in the intestines and cause gas, which in turn can cause painful bloating and cramps. Foods that most often cause gas are the complex carbohydrates such as grains and beans because they are more difficult to digest.

Another consideration is whether you have too much or too little hydrochloric acid (HCI), which helps your stomach digest food. You can test this by putting a tablespoon of apple cider vinegar or lemon juice in a glass of room temperature water and drinking it a half hour or so before dinner. If your indigestion disappears, you may need more stomach acid. You've found the cure—keep taking the apple cider vinegar for relief.

Since stomach acid tends to drop as we age, most older people's heartburn problems are not caused by too much acid, but too little. The undigested food that sits in the stomach is more apt to cause heartburn.

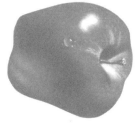

CHAPTER 3

Detoxifying Can Be an Energizing and Illuminating Experience

CHANGE OLD HABITS BY FASTING

YOUR BODY IS ALWAYS DETOXIFYING, every second of every day, but it's easy to overload the system. The most important part of a spring cleaning for the body is cutting way back on food so that your body has a chance to dump accumulated waste and clean itself up.

Fasting in its strictest sense means taking in nothing but water. The early physicians Hippocrates and Paraclesus recommended fasting, and the majority of religions incorporate some type of modified diet or fasting into their rituals. Fasting can be an enlightening experience because it takes us out of our usual context and often, after two or three days, clears the mind.

FASTING WILL CHANGE YOUR POINT OF VIEW ON EATING.

A radical change in eating habits does more than clear the mind and give the body a chance to cleanse and heal itself. It gives you the opportunity to observe your relationship to food. When you reduce your food intake to little or nothing for a few days, you'll notice how much time and energy you devote to thinking about food, shopping for it, preparing and eating it. You'll also notice what foods you're craving, and how automatic it is to walk into the kitchen and open the refrigerator door.

Fasting is a great way to shift into new, healthier eating habits. If you've tried and tried without success to give up or cut down on sweets, chips, coffee, or other harmful foods, a fast can be the perfect opportunity to get the withdrawal symptoms over with and start fresh. If you have arthritis, headaches, fatigue, itchy skin or other symptoms, you may notice they clear up after a few days of fasting. This will be an indication that something you're eating is causing your symptoms, and gives you the opportunity to reintroduce foods one at a time to see which one(s) are causing the symptoms.

GIVE YOUR IMMUNE SYSTEM AND LIVER A BIG BOOST

When we're very sick we often don't want to eat. That can be the body's way of putting all its energy into fighting a disease. Studies show that fasting actually boosts the immune system tremendously, giving it the power to go after a wide variety of toxins ranging from pesticides and bacteria to heavy metals and substances that cause chronic inflammation. Because this effect is so powerful, people who have cancer, autoimmune disease, heart disease, diabetes, or who are recovering from a serious illness, should only fast under the guidance of an experienced health care professional.

Your liver is your primary detoxification factory. During the first few days of a fast your liver may be working hard to dump all the toxins released, but then it will have a wonderful rest period for a few days. Be gentle to yourself and your liver at this time, and avoid any potential sources of toxins or pollution if at all possible. This means avoiding pesticides, air pollution, paint or solvent fumes, new carpeting or furniture, and stress.

PREPARING FOR A FAST

Fasting will go more easily if you prepare yourself. Pick a week when you can spend the week before easing into the fast, and the week after easing off it. Certainly don't pick times when you're traveling or have guests, or times of heavy stress at work. The ideal way to fast is to go to a spa or retreat center with a fasting program, where you can be in a restful, meditative, supportive atmosphere, but I know people who fast while they work full-time, so don't let that stop you.

You can prepare your body for a fast by cutting out or cutting down on meat, fried and fatty foods, and refined grains and sugar. You can also take a detoxifying herbal formula, which will act as a mild laxative, be soothing to the intestine, support your liver, and stimulate your liver and kidneys to pick up the pace of detoxification. By starting a mild detoxification program a week ahead of fasting, you can lessen some of the symptoms of detoxification.

HOW TO DETOXIFY

I'm not a big fan of strict water fasts unless you're under the supervision of a health care professional who is experienced in overseeing them and strongly advocates them. They can induce a rapid detoxification process that can be too harsh.

Depending on your state of health, the first few days of a detoxification process can be very difficult or just mildly uncomfortable as your body adjusts to not eating. Detoxification symptoms can also be caused by withdrawal from coffee, sugar or alcohol. Sometimes parasites can cause an extreme detoxification reaction. If you suspect you have parasites, it's best to do a parasite cleansing program first.

Possible Symptoms of Toxicity

Heart disease, kidney disease, colitis, indigestion, headaches, irritability, dizziness, depression, fatigue, arthritis, immune suppression, insomnia

Possible Symptoms of Detoxification During Fasting

The most common symptom of detoxification is a headache. Other symptoms include fatigue, dizziness, nausea, bad breath, body odor, nausea, mucus discharge, and achy joints

Fruits to Use During a Juice Fast

Apples, pears, apricots

Vegetables to Use for a Juice Fast

Beets, celery, parsley, zucchini, spinach, kale and carrots (limit to one carrot drink per day)

Vegetables to Avoid during a Juice Fast

Broccoli, cauliflower, Brussels sprouts, cabbage, nightshade family veggies (tomatoes, potatoes, and peppers)

Green Drinks to Use for a Juice Fast (One Drink Per Day)

Spirulina, chlorella, or blue-green algae

Vegetables to Use for Steaming on a Modified Fast

Beets, celery, parsley, zucchini, spinach, carrots, broccoli, cauliflower, Brussels sprouts, cabbage, kale, onion, garlic

Grains to Use for a Modified Fast (Rotate Them)

Brown rice, millet, quinoa

Detoxifying and Supportive Herbs

Garlic: blood cleanser, kills parasite and "bad bacteria"

Echinacea: Lymph cleanser, immunostimulant

Licorice root: Called the "great detoxifier" by the Chinese, has some laxative action

Burdock root: Blood cleanser, supports liver, is antibacterial

Oregon grape root: Colon cleanser, blood purifier, supports liver

Yellow dock: Skin and blood cleanser, supports liver, some laxative action

Cascara sagrada: Laxative and bowel cleanser

Dandelion, parsley, and uva ursi: Diuretics that help flush the kidneys and clear the skin

Cayenne and ginger root: Stimulates sweating

Slippery elm bark and fennel: Soothing to mucous membranes

Milk thistle: Supports the liver

Most people do best on a juice fast with psyllium powder, which I'll explain in detail. If you're fasting on your own, it should last a minimum of three days and a maximum of five days.

While you're fasting, don't take any supplements or medications (check with your doctor regarding prescription medications), and of course no coffee, tea or alcohol. If you're on medication and it could threaten your life to go off it, fast with the supervision of a health care professional, so you can safely take your medication while you detoxify. This includes heart disease drugs, insulin, thyroid and steroids. It's OK to keep taking hormone replacement drugs, though I hope you opt for natural options here.

A juice fast can be done with just apple or pear juice three times a day and water, or with the addition of a variety of vegetable juices and green drinks. You want to avoid having fruit juice more than three times a day because it's very sweet and when you stop the fast you'll crave sweets. You also want to encourage your body to burn fat during the fast, and if you're eating too much sugar you'll never get to that point.

It's best to dilute the juice 50/50 with clean water. Of course, I want you to drink 6 to 8 glasses of clean water, in addition to the fruit and vegetable juice, which means you'll probably be sipping something all day. However, remember that the idea isn't to drink so much juice that you feel as full as you would eating normally.

It's best to do a fast in warm weather, because you'll tend to get cold when you're not eating. If you get cold, drink warm, mild herb teas such as chamomile and peppermint. If it's the middle of winter you may want to add a bowl of plain miso soup at lunch.

One of the biggest challenges for people fasting has been getting the intestines working again afterwards. When you stop putting bulk into the intestines, they stop the wave-like motion that moves food through. One solution is enemas. I don't know about you, but I consider enemas an unpleasant experience. However, if you are on a professionally supervised cleansing diet for cancer, I recommend you use enemas.

For everyone else, the problem can be solved by taking psyllium powder during the fast. This provides a neutral source of bulk for the intestines, without doing the work of actual digestion. With your apple or pear juice, mix a tablespoon of psyllium powder and follow that with a glass of room temperature water.

AFTER YOUR FAST

It's often been repeated in the literature on fasting that how you come off a fast is just as important as the fast itself. If you dive right back into your old eating habits, you'll be worse off than when you began. Come off a fast by introducing foods very gradually back into your diet.

I like to break a fast in the morning with an organic baked apple. I follow that with a *small* portion of steamed vegetables (carrots, broccoli, zucchini, spinach) for lunch, and for dinner, I'll have a small salad with olive oil, lemon juice, and salt. The following day I add sprouted whole grain toast with butter to breakfast, steamed brown rice with olive oil to lunch, and a piece of fish or tofu to dinner. You can vary this according to your own tastes, but be gradual and keep portions very small for a few days. Some people don't digest legumes and whole grains very well, so if you fall into that category, introduce them back into your diet very gradually.

A MODIFIED FAST

If a juice fast is too much for you, you can try a modified fast of steamed fresh vegetables and a neutral grain such as rice or millet. I don't recommend eating fruit on this type of fast, because your body will get enough glucose from the carbohydrates provided by the rice and vegetables. You can use a little bit of soy sauce or Bragg's Amino Acids for flavoring, but for best results, eat them plain.

CHAPTER 4

The Double Whammy

SUGAR AND OBESITY

Open sores that were slow to heal repeatedly festered on Teresa's feet. After a number of visits to conventional doctors over the years, one physician finally diagnosed her with type 2 (adult-onset) diabetes, a diagnosis that previous doctors had missed. Not quite understanding the seriousness of her condition, Teresa, now 55, delayed facing her diabetes head on. She began to lose feeling in her feet, so much so that she couldn't step on the brake or the accelerator without first looking to see where her foot was. Confronted with the possibility of amputation, she finally signed up for treatment.

This may sound like an extreme example, but it's not. As many as half of all Americans who have type 2 diabetes go undiagnosed. Early diagnosis is critical because untreated diabetics are at significantly increased risk for coronary heart disease, stroke, and the side effects of peripheral vascular disease, such as the development of foot ulcers. Retinopathy, a disorder of the retina in the eye, can begin within seven years after a person has developed type 2 diabetes if they haven't begun treating it. Thus, early detection and early treatment can reduce the burden of type 2 diabetes and its complications.

Doctors should not have missed Teresa's early warning signs. She had always been a good hundred pounds overweight or more, which she carried predominantly in the stomach, and her blood pressure and cholesterol were always high, although within the "normal" range. Her incredible thirst kept her up all night with frequent trips to the bathroom, and she was always hungry. Furthermore, doctors had suspected that Teresa's own mother had undiagnosed type 2 diabetes, and her father had died of a heart attack, which is one result of the same syndrome that causes diabetes.

With diet and exercise, Teresa has already begun to control her diabetes, but she's not out of the woods for heart disease and other complications. Why is that? Because the medications and the diet (low fat, low protein, high carbohydrates) usually prescribed to type 2 diabetes patients actually creates a vicious cycle of increased glucose levels, which increases insulin levels. Excessive insulin can be just as dangerous as excessive glucose. Conventional medicine is just starting to catch on to the fact that refined carbohydrates such as white bread and white rice raise glucose levels almost as much as white sugar does.

I'll explain about insulin and glucose later, but first I'd like you to meet Roberto. Roberto is not a diabetic, but faces many of the same concerns that trouble Teresa. Despite the low-calorie, low-fat, high-carbohydrate diet prescribed by most public health authorities, Roberto, in his mid-40s, could not lose weight. As a matter of fact, year after year he continued to gain another few pounds and another inch or so around the middle. What's more, he was usually "bone tired," irritable, and had difficulty concentrating. His cholesterol, blood pressure, and triglyceride (blood fat) levels were normal, and because he did not have a family history of diabetes, doctors dismissed diabetes as a health issue.

It is likely that Roberto was insulin resistant, meaning that his insulin was no longer effective in controlling his blood sugar and was, therefore, contributing to his weight gain and other symptoms. Once people become resistant to their insulin, they usually develop insulin resistance syndrome, or Syndrome X, which can cause serious health problems well before type 2 diabetes develops. Syndrome X is a cluster of conditions that include obesity, high cholesterol, high blood pressure, and high triglycerides. The syndrome can lead to type 2 diabetes, circulatory problems, and heart disease.

Although Roberto may never develop type 2 diabetes, he has much in common with Teresa; they each have problematic lifestyles. Mounting evidence shows that a low-fat, high-carbohydrate diet may actually cause weight gain in certain people. This diet may also contribute to glucose intolerance (caused by high blood sugar levels), which develops into insulin resistance syndrome, and ultimately leads to diabetes, hypertension, stroke, and heart failure. It is all part of a continuum that is driven by the delicate balance between glucose (blood sugar) and the hormone insulin.

Genes play a role in developing insulin resistance and type 2 diabetes. Diet and a sedentary lifestyle builds on the foundation that genetics has set down. Your physician might prescribe medications to bring glucose and insulin levels into balance. However, more and more scientifically conducted studies are proving that diet and exercise, aided by vitamin and mineral supplements, can prevent insulin resistance and often reverse type 2 diabetes—with very little or no medication. Even if you are not prone to type 2 diabetes, or even insulin resistance, adjusting your carbohydrate and protein intake can dramatically improve your health and energy.

LET'S LOOK AT THE MATH

It is estimated that 22.4 million Americans have type 2 diabetes, and 65 million Americans are insulin resistant. Diabetes is widely recognized as one of the leading causes of death and disability in the United States. Again, about half of all diabetics are unaware of their condition and therefore are not undergoing treatment. Once thought of as an adult-onset disease (latent until mid-forties), type 2 diabetes is becoming one of the most common chronic disorders in obese and inactive children in the United States.

Prescription drug and medical supply companies consider diabetes quite a profitable market in the United States. In 2007 medical costs for diabetes care, including hospitalizations, medical care and treatment, totaled $174 billion. Indirect costs, including disability payments, time lost from work, and premature death, totaled an additional $54 billion. But it doesn't have to be that way—the cost of changing your diet is minimal.

GLUCOSE AND INSULIN, THE DYNAMIC DUO

Insulin resistance and diabetes are disorders of metabolism—the way in which the body uses digested food for growth and energy. The healthy body converts three kinds of foods into fuels: proteins, fats, and carbohydrates. Proteins, such as dairy products, meats, fish, or eggs, are broken down into amino acids. Fats such as butter, cream, bacon, and oils are broken down into fatty acids. Carbohydrates—whether from cakes, candy, fruits, potatoes, grains or starchy vegetables—are broken down by the digestive juices into simple sugars. Once the sugars enter the bloodstream they are called glucose, a main source of fuel for the body.

After a meal, enzymes secreted by the pancreas go to work directly on the food in the small intestines to break it down and digest it. Glucose passes into the bloodstream where it is available for body cells to use for growth and energy. The pancreas meanwhile also secretes the hormone insulin into the bloodstream. By transporting glucose out of the bloodstream and into the cells, insulin keeps the blood glucose level from rising too high and keeps the cells supplied with fuel.

If you eat nothing for six or eight hours after a meal, your glucose level gradually falls. As it does, the amount of insulin in the blood also falls. When the blood glucose and insulin levels become low, the body tissues— liver, muscle, and especially fat—respond by breaking down storage fuels to produce more glucose. As it enters the bloodstream, glucose stimulates the pancreas to release a little more insulin, which halts the storage fuel breakdown. In this way, the glucose level in the blood is kept within a narrow range.

DIABETES MELLITUS, A TASTE OF HONEY

First described on a 1500 BC Egyptian papyrus, diabetes received its modern name from the Greek word meaning "a siphon" referring to the frequent urination experienced by those with the disease. It is more than a little ironic that the people who first recorded diabetes were witnessing an epidemic within their own culture. Researchers have determined from mummies that their diabetes may have been caused by a high-carbohydrate diet.

The Greek physician Aretus wrote in the second century AD, "The fluid does not remain in the body, but uses the body as a ladder to leave it." This siphoning off, or "melting down of the flesh and limbs into urine," as he described it, often began without warning in children and young people. Besides frequent urination, scribes noted that the disease caused an insatiable thirst, and drinking rivers of water was powerless in preventing water loss, coma, and death.

It was also noted that the patient's urine was typically honey sweet, hence "mellitus" was appended to the name, and until the mid-1800s, tasting the urine was exactly how diabetes was diagnosed. Diabetes mellitus accurately describes the primary symptom, which is the build-up of glucose (blood sugar) in the body, but confuses the symptom for the cause. The major characteristic of diabetes is the body's insensitivity to its own insulin, which regulates the level of glucose in the blood.

Only sixty or seventy years ago, physicians believed that all diabetics were the same because they had the same sweetness of urine—they just suffered from varying degrees of severity. Some got sick in childhood or young adulthood and died following a rapidly progressive illness that was unresponsive to treatment. Others got sick later in life, although never quite as sick, and they seemed to do better on a special diet.

Today, the health community separates diabetes into two broad categories: type 1 (juvenile diabetes), and type 2 (adult-onset diabetes). (A third category, gestational diabetes, develops during pregnancy, and isn't addressed in this book.) Both type 1 and 2 diabetes produce the same imbalance of the body's use of fuel, but for different reasons. More about Syndrome X later, but first, let's look at how a person develops diabetes and further complications.

INSULIN RESISTANCE—PRELUDE TO DISEASE

Insulin was first discovered in 1923 and scientists quickly learned how to use it to help those who could not make their own insulin. Now, three-quarters of a century later, we know that too much insulin can be just as dangerous as too little. Insulin is produced in the pancreas and released into the blood, where it binds to insulin receptors on the surface of cells. Researchers estimate that there are as many as 20,000 insulin receptors or more per cell. Inside the insulin receptor is an enzyme called tyrosine kinase (TK). Once activated by insulin, this enzyme triggers a cascade of events that opens channels through which glucose can enter the cells to be stored or used for energy. When cells become insulin resistant, the channels do not open and the glucose fails to gain entry into the cells. Glucose then builds up in the bloodstream, which in turn signals the pancreas to make more insulin.

Left unchecked, excess glucose flows out from the kidneys (two organs that filter wastes from the bloodstream) into the urine. The glucose takes water with it, which causes frequent urination and extreme thirst. These two conditions—frequent urination and unusual thirst—are usually the first noticeable signs of full-blown diabetes.

TYPE 2 OR ADULT ONSET DIABETES.

In type 2 diabetes, the pancreas still manufactures and releases insulin as fuels arrive. This is enough to move fuel into cells, but the amount of insulin is either insufficient or ineffective, and blood glucose levels tend to rise sharply.

Outdated medical books state that diabetics tend to build up a higher than normal level of sugar, or glucose, in the blood because they lack the proper amount of insulin. It is now known that the reason for the build-up of glucose is that the cells—from a combination of genetics, diet, lifestyle, and almost always, obesity—stop being receptive to insulin's signals to let the glucose in. The pancreas does its best to keep up with the demand by secreting excess levels of insulin to escort glucose into the cells, and the result is chronically high insulin levels.

Type 2 diabetes eventually develops when the pancreas loses the battle, leaving so much glucose in the bloodstream that it begins entering the cells by sheer force. The adult-onset diabetic also frequently loses glucose in the urine, leading to the classic symptoms of excess urination and thirst.

Type 2 diabetes can advance into long-term complications that affect almost every major part of the body, and can lead to blindness, strokes, kidney failure, amputations, and nerve damage. Long-term complications of diabetes include retinopathy with potential loss of vision and nephropathy leading to renal (kidney) failure; peripheral neuropathy (numbness of the extremities) with the risk of foot ulcers and amputation; and other types of neuropathy which cause problems in the digestive tract, the reproductive organs (with resulting sexual dysfunction), and heart disease.

High blood pressure (hypertension), abnormalities of fat metabolism, and gum disease are often found in people with diabetes. Finally, the emotional and social impact of diabetes and the demands of therapy may cause significant emotional and social dysfunction in patients and their families.

INSULIN RESISTANCE SYNDROME, OR SYNDROME X

Imagine the body's cells as little fuel-generating plants that run on sugar, or glucose. Insulin is the plant operator that flips the switch at exactly the right time to allow glucose to be pumped into the cells and converted into energy. Because of its molecular makeup, glucose needs insulin for gentle entry into the cell. Increases in glucose in turn increase the need for insulin. But the cells can take in only so much glucose, and eventually go on strike against the insulin. When this happens, glucose tries to break the dams. What we end up with is an army of insulin plant operators who, in their attempt to bail out buckets of blood sugar, trample and rip up the lining of the arteries.

Insulin resistance syndrome was first observed in the famous Framingham Study, which has followed more than 5,000 men and women since 1949 for signs of heart disease. The study determined that certain risk factors for heart disease tend to cluster, and that insulin resistance and diabetes may be fundamental to this clustering. This constellation of symptoms may cause as much as 25 percent of the cardiovascular disease seen in men and 60 percent of that seen in women.

An overt symptom of insulin resistance syndrome is obesity, especially weight over the belt, or pot belly, as opposed to weight around the hips. Other indications show up on blood tests, including above-normal cholesterol levels, and higher readings on glucose tests commonly used to check for diabetes. People with insulin resistance syndrome may also have elevated blood pressure.

At the center of all these signs and symptoms is a growing inability to use insulin. Muscles become weak and weight gain follows. The continued secretion of insulin promotes the formation of fat (lipogenesis). Without regular physical activity, which burns glucose and lowers insulin levels, insulin keeps increasing the ratio of fat cells to muscle cells. With more fat cells and fewer muscle cells, the body loses still more of its ability to efficiently burn up glucose.

Cholesterol changes linked to insulin resistance can lead to clogged arteries and heart disease. Too much insulin in your blood increases your heart attack risk even if your level of "bad" LDL cholesterol is low. Insulin has that effect on your heart risk because it:

- Raises the level of a type of fat called triglycerides, in your blood.
- Increases the time it takes your body to clear dietary fats from your blood after a meal.
- Lowers your "good" HDL cholesterol.
- Increases your blood's clotting ability.
- Raises your blood pressure.
- Makes particles of "bad" LDL cholesterol smaller and denser.

Syndrome X was first coined in 1968 by a group of researchers at Stanford University who discovered that insulin's ability to do its job varies between people—some were capable of producing enough insulin to compensate for high levels of glucose, while others weren't. Sensitivity to insulin can vary by as much as a factor of ten. The higher levels of insulin that result from insulin resistance cause the liver to increase its production of triglyceride-rich VLDL (Very Low-Density Lipoprotein) and release it into the bloodstream, which increases the risk of coronary heart disease.

The more sugars and carbohydrates an insulin-resistant person eats, the more insulin the pancreas must secrete to prevent the blood glucose from climbing too high. The higher the blood insulin levels, the greater the production of VLDL, and the more the triglyceride levels rise.

OBESITY AND INSULIN RESISTANCE

Not every obese person is insulin resistant, and not all slender people are insulin sensitive. But abdominal obesity plays a key role in insulin resistance, and greatly increases the likelihood of developing manifestations of Syndrome X. Insulin resistance is associated not with the total amount of excess fat, but with how much of it is located in the abdominal cavity, called centralized fat or visceral obesity. Visceral obesity does not necessarily cause high total cholesterol levels, but, rather, is associated with 20 to 25 percent elevations of a specific type of fat component called apo-B, which is an excellent predictor of ischemic heart disease (in which blood supply to the heart is obstructed), and is present in those with insulin resistance syndrome. The combination of high insulin levels and high apo-B as seen in insulin resistance syndrome, increases the risk of heart disease eleven-fold.

GENETICS

Insulin instructs certain cells to open their doors to glucose through a "signal transduction mechanism" involving carrier proteins called GLUT 4 transporters. This complex multi-step process is guided by many genes. Abnormality in one or more of these genes can cause insulin resistance, or a predisposition to insulin resistance. It isn't certain which genes are involved, or if the genes that are at fault are the same from person to person.

Diabetes itself does cluster around certain factors. People who have family members with diabetes (especially type 2 diabetes), who are overweight, or who are African American, Hispanic, or Native American are all at greater risk of developing diabetes.

Type 1 diabetes occurs equally among males and females, but is more common in Caucasians. Data from the World Health Organization's Multinational Project for Childhood Diabetes indicate that type 1 diabetes is rare in most Asian, African, and American Indian populations. Some northern European countries, including Finland and Sweden, have high rates of type 1 diabetes. The reasons for these differences are not known.

Are Your Prescription Drugs Causing Your High Blood Sugar?

How many people have been put on a prescription drug, only to have it cause high blood sugar, precipitating an incorrect diagnosis of diabetes from a doctor, and a prescription for diabetes drugs? Here are some prescription drugs that can cause hyperglycemia, or high blood sugar.

Calcium channel blockers for heart arrhythmias [e.g. nifedipine (Procardia), nicardipine (Cardene), dilitiazem (Cardizem), verapamil]

Antihypertensives that lower blood pressure (e.g. clonidine, diazoixde, diuretics)

Corticosteroids (e.g. Prednisone)

Epinephrine (e.g. bronchodilators, decongestants)

Heparin to prevent blood clotting

Hypothyroid drugs for low thyroid (e.g. Levoxine, Synthroid)

Morphine

Nicotine

Pentamidine for treatment of pneumonia

Phenytoin for the treatment of seizures (e.g. Dilantin)

Antituberculosis drugs [e.g. rifampin (Rifadin, Rimactane), isoniazid (Laniazid, Nydrazid)]

What Is Causing Your Low Blood Sugar?

If you are diabetic, or your blood sugar is unstable, and you are suffering from hypoglycemia or hyperglycemia, you should be aware of those substances that lower your blood sugar:

Alcohol

Allopurinol (e.g.Lopurin, Zyloprim)

Bromocriptine

Chloramphenicol (e.g. Chloromycetin)

Clofibrate (e.g. Abitrate, Atromid-S)

Fenfluramine (e.g.Pondimin)

Indomethacin

Lithium

Mebendazole

Monoamine oxidase inhibitors

Phenylbutazone (e.g. Butatab, Butazolidin)

Probenecid (e.g. Benemid, Probalan)

Salicylates

Sulbactam/ampicillin

Sulfonamides

Tetracycline

Theophylline

NOW, THE GOOD NEWS

The good news about type 2 diabetes and insulin resistance syndrome is that they can be prevented, managed, and frequently even reversed with diet and exercise. If it is true that a high carbohydrate diet of the refined grains found in breads and cereals, refined sugars and other starches can cause an overdose of glucose, which in turn causes high insulin levels, then it is true that cutting back on these food items can help bring them into control.

The ratio of carbohydrates to protein in the diet is much debated in all sectors of the health care fields these days. Because of carbohydrates' effect on insulin and weight gain, a number of diet books advocate eating a low-carbohydrate, high-protein diet to lower insulin, inches, and pounds. On the other hand, replacing carbohydrates with too much protein, while promoting weight loss, may promote kidney damage, may not necessarily reduce the other symptoms of Syndrome X, and may just be a trade-off in the long run.

An old concept is re-emerging, now grounded by sound research: moderation, moderation, moderation! Here's the basic concept: Consume moderate portions of carbohydrates mostly in the form of fresh vegetables, whole grains, nuts, and seeds; slightly smaller portions of high-quality protein, and "good" fats (monounsaturated and fish oil). Studies have shown that just the *attempt* to follow a lower-calorie, balanced diet significantly lowers blood and glucose levels even before the pounds are shed.

With diet and exercise, it is often not necessary to go on the prescription drugs that conventional doctors typically give patients. Remember, the drugs have side effects and over time often make your condition worse, rather than better.

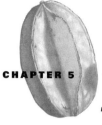

CHAPTER 5

The Achilles' Heel
of the Modern Diet

SUGAR, CARBOHY-DRATES, & BLOOD SUGAR

SANDRA WAS CONSCIENTIOUS WHEN IT CAME TO HER DIET—she worked hard to follow the guidelines that she saw on TV and read about in her women's magazines for healthy eating. She gave up red meat, and high-fat foods such as ice cream. For breakfast she had low-fat bagels with margarine and low-fat cream cheese, and a glass of orange juice. Although she didn't like vegetables very much, she tried to include them in her diet, being sure to include lettuce and even tomatoes on her lunch sandwich that included low-fat bread, low-fat American cheese slices, and low-fat mayonnaise. For dinner she often had chicken wrapped in a white flour tortilla, and included lettuce and tomato there, too. For dessert she would have one cookie—a low-fat brand.

Although Sandra's diet is "correct" according to the advice doled out by TV and magazines (which are supported by processed-food advertisers), it's a nightmare when it comes to maintaining good health. It contains little high-quality protein, almost no quality fat, virtually no fiber, very little in the way of nutrient-dense fruits and vegetables, and is extremely high in refined carbohydrates. Sandra's diet is a set-up for obesity and blood sugar control problems.

Carbohydrates, protein, and fat: These are the triad of *macro*nutrients your body needs to build muscles, charge up organs and life-sustaining systems, absorb nutrients, and store energy for later use. All three types of food, plus vitamin and mineral *micro*nutrients, are essential for good health.

Being overweight is a disorder of the metabolism, the complex physical and chemical action of breaking down or synthesizing nutrients that are vital to maintain your body. One of the root words for metabolism is ballet, and the steps your body takes to use these three types of food can be compared to a well-orchestrated ballet. Numerous complex control systems are constantly at work converting nutrients from one form to another.

Imagine juggling a lemon, a banana, and a cantaloupe. Assuming that you can juggle, it wouldn't take too much energy, timing, and concentration to keep all three going in the air at once, even if they're not the same size, shape, or weight. But what if you tried juggling a sword, a hot iron, and a grape? You would certainly have to concentrate much more to make sure you used just the right amount of strength and timing to keep each object moving constantly, not to mention avoiding harm to yourself. Your arms would soon tire, you would lose concentration, and the objects would drop to the floor.

Similarly, the systems in your body will start to work against you when, over a period of time, you eat any one food group in quantities that are out of proportion to the rest of your diet. Out of ignorance, politics, or a combination of both, the American Diabetes Association and the American Heart Association have recommended low-fat, low-protein, high-carbohydrate diets for decades, and this has only recently begun to change. Ironically, while this diet has created enormous profits for the processed food industry that churns out low-fat processed foods, it has actually contributed to the development of diabetes and heart disease by emphasizing refined carbohydrates and sugar. At the other end of the spectrum, there are a number of books on the market today that recommend high-protein, low-carbohydrate diets, which may help certain individuals lose weight and become more sensitive to their insulin, but can also lead to heart disease, kidney disorders, and muscle and bone loss.

It may surprise you to know that studies are now demonstrating that a diet of moderate portions of proteins and fibrous, vitamin-packed carbohydrates, enriched with generous portions of the right kind of fat, is the most successful in preventing, controlling, and even reversing diabetes and heart disease.

Carbohydrates, protein, and fat all do different things in the body. The key to creating the proper balance is in understanding what each food does and how each can be used to your advantage. You can use food to build muscle, make your brain feel good, wake yourself up, calm yourself down, or to give you quick energy. More importantly, you can use food as medicine to control insulin, cholesterol, weight, and your mental state. In determining the best diet for you, the key words are balance and timing. Vitamins and trace minerals are also critical to this balance. In the following pages, I will describe each food group and their effects.

Fully 80 to 90 percent of all type 2 diabetics are overweight. Insulin resistance is also a side effect of obesity. Obesity in and of itself does not cause insulin resistance and diabetes; lifestyle, an imbalanced diet, and genetics cause insulin disorders—obesity is a side effect that makes it worse. In the rest of this chapter you will learn that healthy foods are tasty and filling, and promote weight loss. What's more, it is a proven fact that losing just ten or fifteen pounds can begin to reverse insulin resistance.

CARBOHYDRATES

Complex carbohydrates, found in fruits, vegetables, grains, legumes, tubers, nuts and seeds, for example, are a primary source of fuel for your body. They provide an immediate and a time-released energy source because they are easily digested and gradually converted into glucose.

Glucose plays an important role in the functioning of the internal organs, the nervous system, the brain and the muscles. At any given time the blood can carry about an hour's supply of glucose. Any glucose that is not needed for immediate energy is converted into glycogen and stored in the liver and muscles. When it is required for energy, the liver turns the glycogen back into glucose. The body can store only enough glycogen to last for several hours of moderate activity.

Some carbohydrates, like a piece of white bread or donut, convert quickly into glucose—too quickly. Anyone eating too much of these foods effectively overdoses on glucose. Because large amounts of glucose are toxic to the kidneys and other organs, the pancreas responds by releasing large amounts of insulin to lower the glucose levels. In turn, the excess insulin wreaks havoc on the body.

If you consume higher levels of carbohydrates than are immediately needed or can be converted to glycogen, then the liver will convert the excess into fatty acids and triglycerides that can be stored as body fat. This process is called lipogenesis. With decreased carbohydrate intake and increased activity levels, fat reserves are converted back to fatty acids for body fuel, a process called lipolysis. Lipogenesis promotes weight gain and lipolysis promotes weight loss.

Some people are genetically engineered to forever be sensitive to excessive amounts of insulin when carbohydrates are consumed in excess. If carbohydrates are consumed in high quantities on a regular basis by a person with a sedentary lifestyle, who is genetically predisposed to becoming resistant to their insulin, weight gain will occur. A particularly hefty combination is large quantities of starchy high-fat food fried in oil. The starch will convert into a flood of glucose, which sets off an alarm for an equal amount of insulin. Fat makes cells more receptive to insulin, and it is also denser in calories. With the gates open, the glucose train slams fat into the cells.

Fat *can* be used advantageously to lower insulin levels and set your body up for allowing the pounds to melt away. Later in the chapter I'll explain why not all fats are created equal, and how eating the right fats can actually help you lose weight. For now, it is important to understand the role of carbohydrates in good nutrition.

COMING FULL CIRCLE WITH CARBOHYDRATES

Our ancestors, like all mammals, ate a relatively simple, yet diverse diet. Carbohydrates were tough, fibrous, and only partially digestible, which promoted a slow, steady increase in glucose and insulin levels. The hunter-gatherer diet did not include mashed potatoes and steamed white rice.

In industrialized countries, particularly in urban areas, there has been a shift away from the healthful consumption of such carbohydrates as fresh fruits, vegetables, whole grains, legumes, and lentils, toward a diet of more refined carbohydrates (white flour, white rice) and simple sugars (table sugar, honey, and fruit). Studies have shown that indigenous peoples around the world and in the United States who move away from their traditional diet toward a diet that is packed with excess calories top-heavy with high-carbohydrate processed foods tend to become obese and develop Western diseases such as heart disease and diabetes.

Until the 1970s, there was an implicit understanding that if we wanted to lose weight, we needed to cut back on starches such as potatoes, bread, cake, and pasta. Then came the McGovern Report in 1977, which encouraged consumption of "complex carbohydrates." The report coined the term to distinguish sugars from whole grains and starches, but it became meaningless when used to describe fruits and vegetables, which are low in starch, but nonetheless carbohydrates. Complex carbohydrates, over the years, have come to describe both the starches that are easily digested and absorbed, and fibers that are not rapidly digested or easily absorbed.

A series of studies in the 1970s from various research groups showed that a diet that included 60 percent carbohydrates actually improved glycemic control and reduced levels of "bad" LDL cholesterol. Researchers observed that people in societies that traditionally consumed a high-carbohydrate diet also had low rates of certain types of heart disease. Together, these findings led some diabetes and heart organizations to recommend a change from the traditional low-carbohydrate diet to a high-carbohydrate diet, although the latter included glucose-spiking pasta, breads, cereals, potatoes, and rice.

Most of us grew up on four basic food groups, which included meat and dairy, starch, fruit, and vegetables. This meal plan was reshaped into the USDA food pyramid, with starchy foods making up the base at six to eleven servings a day. The American Diabetes Association (ADA) acknowledged that carbohydrates would raise your blood glucose more quickly than meats and fats. As a remedy they suggested that your doctor should adjust your medications when you eat more carbohydrates! Why increase medication in order to eat more of the very substance that is causing the condition in the first place? The ADA has begun to back off this misguided advice, but not before contributing to ill health in millions of people.

Building on the "complex carbohydrate" enlightenment of the 1970s, marathoners in the 1980s discovered that eating carbohydrates, like spaghetti and potatoes, gave them extra energy. Somehow we got the notion that if we ate pasta by the wheelbarrowful, we could look as emaciated as a marathoner—without actually running the 26 miles. What's more, we thought that carboloading was healthy. At the same time, we were being told that eggs, red meat, and fat, especially saturated fat, were bad for us because they gave us high cholesterol, opening up a profitable market for low-fat, highly processed foods high in flimsy carbs, hidden sugars, and the wrong kind of oils—all of which promote diabetes and heart disease.

Great Grains: Amaranth

You thought if you cut down on the meat and potatoes you'd be stuck with rice and veggies? No way! I'm going to introduce you to a great grain that really isn't a grain: amaranth. The Aztecs revered amaranth and depended on it for their well-being, so much so that Cortez was reportedly able to conquer them by forbidding the cultivation of this sacred plant.

This nutty-flavored and nutritious treat from Central America is made from the seeds of a broad-leaved plant. It cooks like a grain, is high in protein, and blends well with other grains. Amaranth is higher in protein than any other "grain" except quinoa. Just ½ cup cooked has 14 to 16 grams of protein (nearly half an adult's daily requirement), 7 grams of fat, 150 milligrams of calcium (more than milk plus a much better calcium to magnesium ratio than milk), 266 milligrams of magnesium, 49 micrograms of folacin, and 366 milligrams of potassium. Amaranth is high in the amino acid lysine, which is missing from most grains.

Amaranth grains are about the size of a poppy seed, with a nutty flavor of gelatinous texture when cooked. Since Americans tend not to be partial to gelatinous textures in their grains, many people combine amaranth with other grains such as wheat, barley or rice, which also creates a complete protein. Its texture makes it the perfect thickener for soups and stews.

For a nourishing and warming winter treat, try whole kernel amaranth as a hot breakfast cereal mixed with fruit.

Quinoa, the Mother Grain

This "super food," (pronounced keen-wa) has been a staple in the diet of many native South Americans for centuries. The Incas thought so highly of it they named it the "mother grain." Although it looks, cooks, and taste like a grain, quinoa is not a grain at all—it's actually the dried fruit of an herb. Quinoa is unusual in that it is rich in all eight essential amino acids that compose a "complete protein," and are normally found only in red meat, eggs, and dairy products. However, quinoa has a decided edge over those other foods in that it's much lower in calories and fat and is abundant in fiber. A one-cup serving of quinoa has 129 calories, 2 grams of fat and 4.6 grams of fiber. It's also an excellent source of potassium and iron, as well as a good source of zinc and B vitamins. It cooks in 10 to 15 minutes and has a mild flavor.

I like quinoa mixed with dash of olive oil, some herbs, and steamed veggies (try onions, garlic, mushrooms, zucchini, red peppers, and carrots). If you want to spice that up, add sesame seeds, sunflower seeds, or almonds and some Bragg's Amino Acids or tamari.

Now conventional medical journals are beginning to acknowledge the fact that a high-carbohydrate diet is detrimental to the health of diabetics, as well as to obese people at risk for heart disease, and to all the rest of us as well. Low-carbohydrate diets, they say, along with weight-reduction regimes and exercise, significantly lower insulin levels. But many popular diet books have taken this advice to extremes and recommend severely restricting carbohydrates. Some go as far as to say carbohydrates weren't necessary in the Paleolithic diet, and they're not necessary to our health now.

But wait a minute. Carbohydrates, in sync with protein and good fat, help to fight infections, promote growth of body tissues such as bones and skin, and lubricate the joints. Cutting carbohydrates from the diet to avoid weight gain and to lower insulin levels is not only impractical, it's not healthy and it's certainly not a moderate approach! Carbs are still needed for energy, fiber, and the vitamins and nutrients they contain. The key is to stick to those carbs that don't spike blood sugar.

Researchers now know that although all carbohydrates convert to glucose, not all carbohydrates are created equal—they do not all have the same effect on blood sugar levels. Some forms of starch are rapidly absorbed and digested and induce a steep rise in glucose levels, while others are just the opposite. Over the past two decades researchers have compiled what is known as the glycemic index (GI) to help in assessing which carbohydrates spike glucose levels the most. With the GI Index, we can begin to return to our dietary roots.

Some Herbs and Foods that Lower Blood Sugar

Fenugreek seeds (Trigonella Foenum-graecum)
  (drink as a tea)

Ginseng

Berries (especially blueberries)

Fish

Garlic

Soybeans

Fresh vegetables, especially broccoli

Onions

GLA oils found in evening primrose oil,
  borage oil, black currant oil, and spirulina

Blueberry leaf tea (Vaccinum myrtillus)

Cinnamon

Some Foods that Raise Blood Sugar

Refined sugar, honey

Any refined grain such as white flour, white rice, etc. (Breads labeled "whole wheat" aren't necessarily healthy. Look for "whole grain" breads.)

Carrots

Potatoes

Processed cereals

Raisins

Spaghetti

Sweet corn

Yams

Oatmeal

Oranges

THE GLYCEMIC INDEX—THE MIDDLE ROAD

Did you know that baked potatoes and even brown rice can spike the blood sugar as much as, if not more than, ice cream and chocolate? In 1981, a researcher named David Jenkins published a paper showing that carbohydrates differ dramatically in how they affect blood sugar. He devised the glycemic index as a means of ranking foods based on their blood glucose-raising potential. The glycemic index ranks foods on how each 50-gram serving affects blood sugar levels two to three hours after eating. Scientists have so far measured the glycemic indexes of about 300 high-carbohydrate foods.

Eating foods that have the least sugar-boosting potential helps keep blood sugar down, and hence less insulin is needed to process them. The chart below will help you determine how much specific foods raise blood sugar. One of your keys to blood sugar balance is to choose foods with the lowest numbers. Generally, foods ranking between 1 and the low 60s only minimally affect blood sugar levels and are therefore preferable. Foods ranking between the low 60s and high 80s are considered moderate and should be eaten in moderation, and foods ranked 90 and above are higher and should be eaten sparingly.

Scientists and dieticians usually base their GI ratings on glucose syrup and white bread, which have a nearly identical GI. In other words, foods scoring higher than 100 increase your blood sugar more than glucose syrup or white bread and those under 100 increase your blood sugar less than glucose syrup or white bread.

I don't want you to turn the GI index into a religion, but you should become familiar with it. Glucose response to a particular food is highly individual, so there are significant differences in response from person to person. The same type of food can also vary tremendously. Potatoes, for instance, can show different measurements depending on the variety, where they are grown, how they are cultivated, and the way in which they are prepared. Also, combinations of foods can produce varied results.

Barley, beans, lentils, yogurt. Sound familiar? These types of foods are eaten frequently in cultures that have low rates of obesity. Some studies suggest that a low GI diet reduces the risk of developing non-insulin dependent diabetes in both men and women. Clinical trials have also shown a decrease in serum triglycerides (blood fats) in normal individuals as well as in those with diabetes and other cardiovascular problems. Since these foods digest more slowly, they aid in the metabolism of fat. Put simply, eating low GI foods will help in losing weight.

FEELING FULL—THE SATIETY INDEX

You know the old joke about eating Chinese food—you'll be hungry again in an hour. That's because rice, like pasta and bread, is moderately easy and quick to digest. Studies by Australian researcher Dr. Susanne Holt and her associates at the University of Sydney show that some carbohydrates curb the appetite more than others. Dr. Holt developed the satiety index (SI) to rank different foods on their ability to satisfy hunger. The index has important implications for those wanting to lose weight.

Using white bread as the baseline of 100, the Holt study scored thirty-eight different foods. In other words, foods scoring higher than 100 are more satisfying than white bread and those under 100 are less satisfying. After eating one specific food, students in the test recorded their feelings of hunger every fifteen minutes, and over the next two hours they could go to a buffet table and eat as much as they liked. All servings were 240-calorie portions.

Dr. Holt found that croissants are only half as satisfying as white bread,

The Glucose Index (White Bread = 100)

BREADS

Barley kernel 49±5

Rye kernel 71±3

Rye flour 92±3

Rye crispbread 93

Barley flour 95±2

White bread 100±0

GRAINS

Pearled barley 36±3

Rye kernels 48±4

Corn tortilla 54

Wheat kernels 59±4

Bulgur 68±3

Rice, parboiled 68±4

Cracked barley 72

Sweet corn 78±2

Specialty rices 78±2

Buckwheat 78±2

Rice, brown 79±6

Rice, white 81±3

Rice, high amylase 83±5

Couscous 93±9

Cornmeal 98±1

Millet 101

Tapioca 115±9

Rice, low amylase 126±4

Rice, instant 128±

CEREAL

All bran 60±7

Oat bran 78±8

Muesli 80±14

Porridge oats 87±2

Shredded wheat 99±9

Puffed wheat 105±3

Cornflakes 119±5

Puffed rice 123±11

FRUIT

Apricots, dried 44±

Bananas, underripe 51

Apples 52±3

Pears 54±4

Apple juice 58±1

Oranges 62±6

Peaches, canned 67±12

Orange juice 74±4

Kiwifruit 75±8

Mangoes 87±7

Bananas, overripe 82±11

Paw paws 83±3

Bananas 83±6 5

Apricots, canned 91

LEGUMES

Soy beans 23±3
Lentils 38±3
Kidney beans 42±6
Lentils, green 42±6
Butter beans 44±3
Split peas, yellow 45
Lima beans 46
Chickpeas 47±2
Haricot beans 54±8

Peas, dried green 56±12
Canned chickpeas 59±1
Black-eyed peas 59±12
Pinto beans 61±3
Peas, green 68±7
Baked beans 69±12
Lentils, green canned 74
Kidney beans, canned 74

PASTA

Spaghetti, brown 53±7
Spaghetti, white 59±4
Other 59±3
Macaroni 64

Linguine 71±4
Spaghetti, durum 78±7
Macaroni, boxed 92

SOUPS

Tomato 54

Bean soups 84±7

ROOT VEGETABLES

Carrots 70
Yams 73
Sweet potatoes 77±11
Beets 91
White potatoes, mashed 100±2
White potatoes, boiled 80±2

New potatoes 81±8
French fries 107
Instant potatoes 118±16
Baked potatoes 121±16
Parsnips 139

DAIRY PRODUCTS

Yogurt 27±7
Milk, whole 39±9
Milk, skim 46
Soy milk 43

Yogurt 48±1
Ice cream 84±9
Frozen tofu 164

BAKED GOODS

Pizza, cheese 86	Cookies 90±3
Cakes 87±5	Crackers, wheat 99±4
Muffins 88±9	Rice cakes 123±6

SNACKS

Peanuts 21±12	Hard candy 100
Potato chips 77±4	Corn chips 105±2
Popcorn 79	Jelly beans 114
Chocolate 84±14	

SUGARS

Fructose 32±2	Sucrose 87±2
Lactose 65±4	Honey 104±21

GI=glycemic index (white bread=100)

± represents the mean average of various studies, plus or minus the range of results.

while potatoes scored highest, and are more than three times as satisfying as white bread. Chips gave almost twice as much satisfaction as doughnuts, and popcorn scored higher than bran cereal.

Theoretically, fatty foods are not satisfying because the body doesn't recognize the fat as energy for immediate use, and so it doesn't tell the brain to cut hunger signals. Carbohydrates, on the other hand, raise blood glucose so the body knows it has enough fuel. Overall, the carbohydrates cut hunger feelings, while protein-rich foods such as cheese, eggs, baked beans, meat, and fish come in second, and fruit third. But there are big differences between the satisfaction value of foods within the same group.

The SI scores only reflect the total amount of fullness produced by the test foods in specific portions over a two-hour period, which is really a short-term satiety. Although most foods with high SI scores kept fullness relatively high for the entire two hours, there were a few exceptions. Servings were kept at 240 calories, and so when it came to fruit, the serving was large and quite filling. But the fullness dropped off quickly toward the end of the second hour as the stomach quickly emptied.

Satiety Index and Glucose Index Comparison Chart

BAKED PRODUCTS	SI RATING	GI RATING
Croissant	47%	96
Cake	65%	87
Doughnuts	68%	108
Cookies	120%	90
Crackers	127%	99

CARBOHYDRATES	SI RATING	GI RATING
White bread	100%	100
French fries	116%	107
White pasta	119%	59
Brown rice	132%	79
White rice	138%	81
Grain bread	154%	69
Brown past	188%	53
Potatoes	323%	77–121

BREAKFAST CEREALS WITH MILK	SI RATING	GI RATING
Muesli	100%	80
Sustain	112%	97
Special K	116%	77
Corn Flakes	118%	119
Honey Smacks	132%	78
All-Bran	151%	60
Porridge/Oatmeal	209%	87

FRUITS	SI RATING	GI RATING
Bananas	118%	83
Grapes	162%	66
Apples	197%	52
Oranges	202%	62

SNACKS	SI RATING	GI RATING
Peanuts	84%	21
Yogurt	88%	27, 48
Potato chips	91%	77
Ice cream	96%	84
Jellybeans	118%	114
Popcorn	154%	79

PROTEIN RICH FOODS	SI RATING	GI RATING
Lentils	133%	42
Cheese	146%	NA
Eggs	150%	NA
Baked beans	168%	69
Beef	176%	NA
Ling fish 225%	NA	

Note: In this chart both SI and GI ratings are compared to white bread, ranked at 100.

BULK FOODS—ALL YOU CAN EAT

One quality that makes a food satisfying is its sheer bulk. For example, you can eat a lot of popcorn without taking in a lot of calories. Popcorn has a moderately high GI rating, but you can eat a few cups and still feel full. Oranges come out very high on the index for the same reason, but the same amount of orange juice without fiber won't make you feel as full. Size, bulk, and the blandness of potatoes may account for much of their high satiety; their portion weight is up to four times greater than other foods with the same caloric content. Boredom has a lot to do with feeling full—you'll satiate quickly on any nearly any food if that's all you eat. That's why you can consume a lot of calories grazing at a buffet or cocktail party.

Chemical compounds in foods also contribute to the feeling of fullness. Beans and lentils, for example, contain substances that delay their absorption so they make you feel full longer. In general, the more fiber, protein, and water a food contains, the longer it will satisfy.

The key is to find foods that have a low GI rating, while making you full at the same time. The following table lists foods that can be eaten safely in bulk to satisfy hunger without worry of excessive calorie intake. Again, don't go overboard with this, just use it to increase your awareness of how you eat.

Examples of Bulk Foods

Apples	Collard Greens	Oranges
Apricots	Eggplant	Peaches
Artichokes	Endive	Peppers, chile
Asparagus	Grapefruit	Pineapples
Bean Sprouts	Lettuce	Plums
Beets	Loquat	Seaweed (wakame)
Blackberries	Melons	Spinach
Broccoli	Mushrooms	Squash
Brussel Sprouts	Mustard greens	Tangerines
Cabbage	Nectarines	Tomatoes
Cantaloup	Oatmeal	Turnips
Cauliflower	Okra	Watercress
Celery	Onions	Zucchini

FIBER

The beneficial effects of fiber appear to have been known since biblical times. Only in recent years have scientist begun to understand its importance in the daily diet as a means of preventing disease and maintaining health. Fiber can be a great ally in weight loss because it gives you the feeling of being full, but doesn't add calories.

The fiber content of foods is important in the bulking of the stool, which aids in regular elimination of waste materials. As fiber passes through the digestive tract, it sponges up many times its own weight in liquid. The result is softer, bulkier stools that pass through the intestine more rapidly, thus decreasing constipation. Some of the soluble fibers such as those found in fruit, oat bran and others, can lower blood cholesterol levels and help to control blood sugar levels because they are slow to digest. I recommend daily consumption of 20 to 35 grams of fiber from a wide variety of high-fiber foods. The typical American diet is estimated to provide about 12 grams of fiber a day.

DIETARY SOURCES OF FIBER

The best dietary fiber comes from fruits, vegetables, beans, peas, cereals, grains, nuts and seeds. The outer layer of a grain, which contains the most fiber, is often removed in the refining process. This explains why whole-grain products such as brown rice and whole-grain bread are such good sources of fiber.

Fiber falls into two broad categories: soluble and insoluble. The soluble fibers dissolve into water and become sticky. They include pectin, available in fruits, nuts, legumes, as well as some vegetables and mucilages, a gummy substance in plant seeds.

Insoluble fiber does not dissolve and passes largely unchanged through the digestive tract in its chewed state. Insoluble fibers include cellulose found in bran, whole grains, and vegetables; hemicelluloses, contained in fruits, nuts, whole grains, and vegetables; and lignin, a woody substance that is also found in bran, nuts, whole grains, and the skins of fruits.

OTHER WAYS OF INCREASING FIBER INTAKE

- Eat the skins of organic potatoes, apples and other fruits, and vegetables.

- Use whole-grain cereals, breads and brown rice; avoid products made from white or highly processed flour.

- If you can't tolerate a particular high-fiber food, substitute something else. For example, replace beans with another vegetable.

- You will need fairly large amounts of high fiber, more than a single serving a day, to reap the benefits you're looking for. Choose four from the following unusually good sources:

High Fiber Foods

FOOD	Serving Size Needed For Fiber Content
Apples	2 medium
Apricots	2 raw, 10 dried
Artichokes	½
Avocado, Califonia	1
Bananas	1½ raw
Beans, kidney	⅓ cup cooked
Beans, lima	¼ cup cooked
Beans, pinto	⅓ cup cooked
Bran cereals	¾ to 1 cups
Broccoli	¾ cup cooked
Cantaloupe	¼
Cauliflower	¾ cup raw
Chickpeas	½ cup cooked
Corn	½ cup
Eggplant	1 cup cooked
Figs	2 medium
Grapefruit, white	½
Greens: collard, kale mustard, turnip	1 cup cooked
Lettuce, dark green	1 cup
Oat bran	⅓ cup dry
Oatmeal	¾ cup cooked
Okra	¾ cup
Peas, cowpeas, blackeyed	¼ cup cooked
Peas, green	½ cup cooked
Peas, split	½ cup cooked
Potato	¾ medium, baked
Prunes	5
Squash, zucchini summer	¾ cup
Strawberries	1 cup
Whole wheat spaghetti	5 ounces
Whole grain bread	1 slice

PSYLLIUM SEED

Psyllium seed husk (pronounced sil-ee-um) is a good source of fiber, especially if you can't bring yourself to consume the recommended 30 grams of fiber a day. You know it as Metamucil (which is loaded with artificial colorings, sugar or NutraSweet). Pure psyllium is better for you and cheaper. All you do is stir a teaspoon to a tablespoon of psyllium into a glass of water or juice and drink. There are capsules you can take if you prefer, but they do not contain as much fiber as the bulk form does. Your health food store may carry psyllium in its bulk section. One tablespoon of psyllium contains 6 to 8 grams of fiber.

TAMING THE COOKIE MONSTER

Cookies are as American as apple pie and McDonalds, but if the cookie monster has got you, it can sabotage a healthy lifestyle. Most supermarket cookies contain at least four of the big no-no's: refined white flour, white sugar, hydrogenated vegetable oils, and a long list of preservatives and additives. But there is a way to have your cookies and eat them too!

If you have kids, your cookie needs will probably differ from that of an adults-only household. Most adults can get along fine with cookies as an occasional treat, but kids seem to require them, along with peanut butter and jelly sandwiches and hamburgers with ketchup. You can satisfy your kids' cookie craving with healthy cookies—just don't tell them they're healthy!

Here's what to look for in a healthy cookie: Whole grain flour, non-hydrogenated vegetable oils, and fruit juice as a sweetener. They are free of refined sugar, and don't have artificial preservatives or food dyes. Look for cookies made with eggs, butter, milk, oats, raisins and other dried fruit, and spices such as cinnamon.

My personal approach to cookies is this: I don't eat them as a regular snack food. It's much healthier to snack on things like fruit, raw vegetables, nuts, and popcorn.

CHAPTER 6

What Does It All Have to Do with Your Weight?

USING PROTEIN TO YOUR ADVANTAGE

WHETHER YOU'RE A FORMER MARINE who used to eat red meat three times a day and still eats it nearly every day, or a slim athlete and vegetarian, you're probably not eating protein in a way that's optimally healthy for you. Myths about protein abound, and the confusion over when and how to eat protein is only matched by the debate over which types of protein are best for you. Plenty of otherwise well-educated people aren't even sure what protein is, and if you fall into that category I'll clear that up shortly.

There is much controversy about whether fat makes you gain weight faster, or sugars and carbohydrates make you gain weight faster. I hate to tell you folks, but bottom line: eating too much is what causes you to gain weight. It doesn't matter whether it's fat, sugar, carbohydrates, or a side of beef—it's the food!

Having said that, it's equally nutritional nonsense to claim that calories are calories are calories, and that the type of calories doesn't matter—of course it does. The body responds much differently to 400 calories worth of fat than it does to 400 calories worth of sugar.

Then why have Americans gained so much on the endless variations of high-carbohydrate, low-fat diets that have been "politically correct" for the past 30 years? One possible explanation is that carbohydrates are a mood enhancer—the more you eat, the more serotonin your brain makes. In other words, there is a marked decrease in anger, depression, and confusion 90 to 180 minutes after eating, say, a bowl of cereal.

Unfortunately, most people don't turn to the carbohydrates that quell hunger when they feel bad, like beans and high-fiber cereals; instead, they turn to chips, white bread, fast food, pasta, and baked potatoes. Rather than a sustained burn, blood sugar levels spike sharply, and an inevitable roller coaster ride of mood ensues. Studies have also shown that this calming factor of carbohydrates doesn't work as well in overweight people.

The medical community is beginning to agree that certain kinds of carbohydrates cause glucose intolerance, insulin resistance, and weight gain, while others reverse these conditions. But carbohydrates complete only one third of the story. Protein is another essential component of nutrition and well-being. However, like carbohydrates, protein is also drawing controversy as to its role in disease and weight loss.

PROTEIN

Protein—found in eggs, meat, fish, legumes, nuts, seeds, grains (in smaller amounts), and dairy products—is essential to the growth and repair of every cell in your body. Protein aids in digestion, immunity, and many other functions. Proteins help form bones and hemoglobin in blood, and help make hair and nails. The antibodies that protect us from disease, the enzymes needed for digestion and metabolism, the insulin and other hormones that regulate energy, are all made of protein. From the amino acid building blocks that you get from protein, your body in turn makes thousands of complex proteins that have innumerable functions in your body. In fact, it's such an inherently valuable nutritional substance that your body will actually recycle some proteins rather than excrete them. A certain amount of protein is lost through normal wear and tear and must be replaced from the diet. But to use this protein, the body must first break it down into individual amino acids and then reassemble them according to the body's genetic code.

In the stomach, chains of amino acids called peptides are broken into shorter chains called polypeptides. Digestion continues in the small intestine, where pancreatic and other enzymes complete the process. The individual amino acids are absorbed into the bloodstream, which carries them to cells. Because amino acids are not stored as such, those that are not used in a relatively short time are returned to the liver, where the nitrogen is removed, and they are sent on to the kidneys to be excreted as urea. The remaining protein molecules are stored as fat or converted to glucose for energy.

GLUCAGON, THE OPPOSING FORCE OF INSULIN

Some amino acids are retained in the liver and converted into glucose by means of a hormone called glucagon. Glucagon, which is produced by the alpha cells in the pancreas when food is eaten, plays a role in glucose management by providing a balancing or opposing effect on insulin. Glucagon keeps the pancreas from making too much insulin and allows the body to burn stored fat and stored carbohydrates (glycogen) for energy. When glucose levels fall, you feel hungry. In order to boost and normalize glucose, glucagon signals the release of glycogen (stored glucose) from the liver, and promotes the conversion of protein into glucose (a process called gluconeogenesis). In this way the pancreas and liver work together to maintain a tightly controlled amount of glucose in the bloodstream at all times.

Without insulin the blood sugar would soar, causing dehydration, coma, and death. On the other hand, the brain requires blood sugar to operate, so an absence of glucagon would allow the blood sugar to fall too rapidly, causing brain dysfunction, coma, and then death.

Excess insulin elevates blood pressure; causes the kidneys to hold on to salt and fluid; promotes growth in the muscular layer of the artery walls, making them thicker and less pliable; increases the level of norepinephrine, an adrenaline-like substance that raises the heart rate and constricts blood vessel; and increases the liver's production of LDL cholesterol. In other words, chronically high insulin is deadly.

Glucagon, on the other hand, sends signals to the kidneys to release excess salt and fluid; the liver to slow down the production of cholesterol and triglycerides; the artery walls to relax and drop blood pressure; and the fat cells to release stored fat to be burned for energy. When insulin levels are too high, glucagon is so overwhelmed, it can't do its job. If insulin is the plant manager that allows the fuel glucose into the little generating plants that are the cells, then glucagon is the foreman. So, what's the problem, you ask? If blood sugar problems are related to an overload of insulin, because of an overload of glucose, why can't glucagon solve the problem?

It all goes back to diet. A high-carbohydrate diet drives the insulin side out of control, but it is protein (along with fat) that primarily stimulates the release of glucagon to control the insulin.

COMING FULL CIRCLE WITH PROTEINS

Hundreds of thousands of years ago, our Paleolithic ancestors gathered a variety of plant foods, and hunted large and small game. It is estimated that protein from meat made up at least 30 percent of their diet (some say 60 to 90 percent). Anthropologists and archaeologists have seen that in groups such as the Eskimos, who for months on end ate almost nothing but protein and fat from whales and other arctic wildlife, there were no cases of diabetes or heart disease.

Humans have been on the planet in one form or another for at least four million years, and evolved genetically during that time primarily as meat eaters. Grains have been a staple of the diet for only about 10,000 years, a very short part of our genetic history and evolution. Even in ancient Egypt, an agrarian society, diabetes and heart disease proliferated.

A century ago, half of all Americans still lived on farms where they raised their own free-range meat without chemicals, hormones, and antibiotics. They fished in fresh water and continued to hunt for game. Their diets still included 30 percent protein, their consumption of refined carbohydrates and sugar was moderate and, thus, insulin resistance and diabetes were rare. Game meats our ancestors ate were higher in muscle and lower in total fat and saturated fat than the meat we eat today. We can compare the Paleolithic meats to modern venison, rabbit, and buffalo. A 100-gram portion of game meat contained 22 grams of protein, and 4 grams of fat. The same portion of domestic meat we buy in the grocery store today consists of 16 grams of protein and 29 grams of fat. What's more, game meats are rich in omega-3 fatty acids, while grocery store meat is high in carbohydrates and omega-6 fatty acids produced when animals aren't exercised and are fed corn instead of grass. Granted, our ancestors highly valued fatty meat, but the supply of it was naturally limited.

Today, we consume more dairy products, and fewer vegetables, nuts, seeds, and fish. Our meats are high in preservatives, such as sugar and salt, and have been exposed to pollutants, hormones, pesticides, and antibiotics.

NOT EATING ENOUGH PROTEIN

People who don't get enough protein tend to suffer deficiencies approaching that of people living in most parts of rural Africa and other underdeveloped areas. There, the dietary staples are starchy protein-deficient foods such as yams, and cassava. Severe protein deficiency (Kwashiorkor) is marked by poor growth and mental impairment in children, edema, anemia, muscle wasting, decreased immunity, and metabolic abnormalities. This state of malnutrition makes these populations highly susceptible to AIDS and other wasting diseases. Furthermore, the overload of insulin unchecked by protein-stimulated glucagon can cause diabetes and a variety of other issues primarily related to the cardiovascular system.

EATING TOO MUCH PROTEIN

Excessive protein that is not balanced by carbohydrates is also bad for your health. An excessively high-protein, no-carbohydrate diet can help you shed pounds, but it can also cause your blood to become too acidic, throw off the mineral balance in your cells, cause a calcium deficiency, and put an unnecessary burden on your kidneys and liver. If you have diabetes or kidney problems it's a good idea to keep your protein intake very balanced with carbohydrates.

Let's look at the pro and cons of eating lots of protein. Protein is acidic, so your kidneys tap into your body's calcium reserves to balance this acidity. If there's not enough calcium in your blood, it will be pulled from your bones. This not only sets you up for osteoporosis, it also throws off the mineral balance in your cells. Metabolizing excess protein, especially without carbohydrates, can put a great strain on your kidneys and liver. Most of the protein in high-protein diets comes from meat, which brings up another risk: Meat—unless it's organic—is contaminated with pesticides, estrogenic drugs and antibiotics.

Let's take a closer look at this process: Extremely high-protein, low-carbohydrate crash diets are "ketogenic" regimens that force the body to turn to protein and stored fat for energy. For the first few days, the body breaks down its lean muscle tissue and converts the protein to glucose. But if this process were allowed to continue, death could occur within weeks. Instead, the body tries to conserve protein by burning fat. Ketones, a byproduct of excessive fat metabolism, build up in the blood, so the kidneys increase urination to get rid of them. Dieters mistake the drop in weight for a loss of fat. In reality, most early weight loss is water, and weight quickly returns when carbohydrates are consumed again. You can also feel tired, irritable, and cranky on a high-protein diet because there is not enough glucose in the blood.

While severe ketosis can be unhealthy, there's another side to it. As Michael and Mary Dan Eades, authors of the book *Protein Power,* explain, a mild state of ketosis can be healthy because ketone bodies are made when fat breaks down. You make them all the time, but unless you're currently on a high-protein diet or have been fasting, you're probably not in ketosis, which is the state of having a measurable level of ketones in your blood. The Eades, who advocate a fairly moderate "high protein" diet, maintain that ketones are not poisonous and are the preferred fuel for the heart.

However, the body must have sufficient amounts of carbohydrates to completely burn all the ketones that are produced for energy. Extremely high-protein diets that cut out almost all carbohydrates don't provide enough carbohydrates to burn off all of the ketones, and since ketones are incompletely burned fat, the body releases them via the stool, the urine, or the breath. We do not recommend that you go to this extreme. There's no reason to stress your body this way.

So what's the answer? Moderation, moderation, moderation! Keep your carbohydrates complex and eat them in moderate amounts. Much of your carbohydrate intake can be in form of fresh vegetables. Eat enough high-quality protein to balance your carbohydrate intake, and don't overeat. Sound simple? It is!

WHEN TO USE A HIGH PROTEIN DIET

If you are insulin resistant, a somewhat high-protein diet can help decrease your risk for heart attack only if you lose excess weight and keep it off by not eating too much and getting some exercise. So, as long as you're in the process of losing weight, eating more protein than usual shouldn't do you any harm. Actively losing weight improves insulin sensitivity and you need less insulin to transfer blood sugar to cells. If you stop losing weight and hold steady, a high-protein diet can actually elevate insulin levels as much as a high-carbohydrate diet. According to Dr. Reaven, this is because while amino acids from protein stimulate the production of glucagon, they also stimulate the production of a little insulin.

All in all, a very high-protein, low-carbohydrate diet is based on playing a trick with your metabolism, and is not a healthy way to lose weight or to eat in the long run. On the other hand, cutting down on carbohydrates and increasing protein is probably a good idea for those with blood sugar imbalances. If you want to follow a higher protein diet for awhile, please read either *Protein Power* by the Eades, or *The Zone* by Barry Sears, both of which advocate a fairly moderate approach to carbohydrate and protein balance. However, unlike these authors, I do not recommend lunch meats or other processed foods, or artificial sweeteners—please stick to whole foods as much as possible.

HOW TO USE PROTEIN TO YOUR ADVANTAGE

Protein is a vital component of your diet. Protein serves many important purposes, and you can use it to your advantage in controlling glucose and insulin, and in losing weight. Protein is a prime source for an amino acid called tyrosine, which increases production of energizing neurotransmitters in the brain. Eating some protein in the morning can help you feel mentally sharp. Avoid eating too much protein at night unless you want to stay alert.

Over a period of many hours, protein subdues hunger pangs more than fat and carbohydrates. If you eat protein by itself or at the beginning of the meal instead of bread or a salad, it will help satiate your appetite. If you include protein such as beef or turkey jerky in snacks, it will help you avoid overeating. People who skip meals tend to overload on carbohydrates at the end of the day, which is not burned off and actually causes weight gain.

How about people who are obese and insulin resistant? Let's face it. The insulin resistant individual is probably at least 20 to 30 pounds overweight, while the type 2 diabetic is likely severely overweight. The best way to prevent or reverse the symptoms is to lose weight, preferably on a diet that doesn't fight you along the way. You don't want to eat too much of the food that is causing your insulin to rise. I've seen the effects of carbohydrates on weight, but how much protein is enough?

If you use protein strategically to satiate hunger, you will automatically eat fewer calories. For most people, 100 calories of protein are needed to satiate hunger. One study fed 155 calories of protein to a group of obese people, who, by the second meal, required fewer calories. They could easily eat 1,000 or more calories as high GI carbohydrates, but found it difficult to consume 700 calories of protein in a day. A very general guideline is to consume between 20 and 30 percent of your calories as protein. The amount of protein that you eat will depend entirely on what works best for you. Keep in mind that everyone is different in their genetics, biochemistry, overall health and lifestyle, so it's impossible to give exact numbers. It may be that more or less works best for you. You need to experiment and find out what balance makes you feel optimally healthy and energetic.

Here's an overview of some sources of protein:

Legumes: Beans are low on the glycemic index, including soy, lentils, and kidney beans. They are a good source of protein, especially when combined with a complex carbohydrate. Avoid canned beans. If beans give you indigestion, try adding them to your diet more gradually. Some people can't eat beans at all because they aren't genetically equipped to digest them. This is particularly true of Caucasians of Northern European descent.

Dairy products: I do not recommend that adults drink milk because most are lactose-intolerant, but unsweetened yogurt, hard cheeses, and eggs are a good source of protein.

Fish: I particularly recommend king or Atlantic salmon, rainbow trout, Atlantic cod, haddock, halibut, mackerel and anchovies—fish which are also rich in omega-3 fats that help to lower insulin levels.

Game meat: Buffalo, rabbit, ostrich, and venison lower cholesterol and are lower in fat and higher in protein.

Other meats: Try eating turkey, chicken, and lean red meat that is baked, broiled, steamed, stewed, sautéed, grilled (but not charred), or poached.

Please avoid eating processed, smoked, and pickled meats such as bologna, hot dogs, and ham as a regular part of your diet. There's nothing wrong with a hot dog now and then, but it's well-proven by now that the preservatives in these types of meats are not good for you.

Virtually all Americans are intimately familiar with the various nuances of buying, preparing and eating meat. While I'm not an advocate of making beans your primary source of protein, you will benefit from becoming better acquainted with them and eating them on a regular basis.

GETTING ALL YOUR ESSENTIAL AMINO ACIDS

Humans require 20 different amino acids. Eleven of these can be supplied by the body, but the other nine, referred to as essential amino acids, must come from the diet. If an essential amino acid is missing from the diet, the body breaks down lean tissue to get it, leading to the muscle wasting over time. Animal protein provides all nine essential amino acids in the proportions required by the human body. Most plant protein lacks one or more of the essential proteins.

The body can build a complete protein from plant foods if they are combined in such a way that they complement each other. For example, grains are high in the essential amino acid methionine, but they lack lysine. Lysine is plentiful in dried beans, peanuts, and other legumes, which are deficient in methionine. By combining a grain with a legume, you can obtain the complete range of amino acids.

Many of the favorite low-meat dishes from non-industrialized countries provide complementary proteins: the beans and corn tortillas of Mexico; the rice and dahl (split peas) of India; the tofu, rice, and vegetable combinations in Asian cuisine; the chickpeas and bulgur wheat in Middle Eastern dishes; and such American favorites as baked beans and corn bread, as well as succotash (lima beans and corn).

THE LOWLY LEGUME: NATURE'S (ALMOST) PERFECT FOOD

I know what you're saying already about beans! "Beans, beans make you toot!" I chanted that rhyme in grade school too. Yes, beans can give you gas, but I'll tell you how to solve that problem. First, let's take a look at why I think beans are one of nature's perfect foods.

- **Beans** are a great source of plant protein.
- **Beans** are high in fiber, 5 to 9 grams of fiber per cooked cup, and the high fiber content helps lower cholesterol and prevent colon cancer.
- **Beans** are low in fat.
- **Beans** are low in calories.
- **Beans** are low in sodium.
- **Beans** contain complex carbohydrates, which cause a gentle rise in blood sugar.
- **Beans** are a good source of B vitamins, zinc, potassium, magnesium, calcium, and iron.

So, why do beans give us gas? Because they contain complex sugars called oligosaccharides that are not easily broken down by the digestive system. When these sugars reach the colon undigested, the bacteria there chow down on them and a by-product of this digestive process is gas. There are a number of ways to avoid giving your colon bacteria a gas-producing feast.

One of the reasons people don't digest beans well is that their digestive systems don't contain the necessary enzymes to break down the sugars, starches, and fiber in beans. However, your body is remarkably intelligent, and if you introduce new foods into your diet gradually, your body will make the needed enzymes. Most people eat a big meal of beans, find them indigestible, and rarely try them again. Try eating just ¼ to ½ cup at first, perhaps mixed with rice or in a soup. Do this a few times a week for two or three weeks, and then try eating more.

A third alternative is to introduce your digestive system to the needed enzymes by using a product called Beano which is now found in your local health food store and in many pharmacies and supermarkets. Beano contains an enzyme called alpha-galactosidase, which will help break down those pesky sugars. A drop or two of Beano on a serving of beans should eliminate most if not all of the gas problems.

One of the simplest ways to eliminate the gassy sugars is to pre-soak the beans. This, in effect, releases the complex sugars and pre-digests the beans. The best way to soak beans is overnight. Since they expand to two to three times their dry size, put them in a large bowl and cover them with water. Before you cook the beans, throw away the soaking water and add new water.

Although I haven't tried this, I've heard that adding a little bit of apple cider vinegar to the beans in their last stages of cooking helps break down the indigestible sugars. Some cultures add fennel to the beans to aid in their digestion, and in Mexico, cumin is often added.

THESE ARE A FEW OF MY FAVORITE BEANS

Soybeans, should be eaten primarily in their fermented form, which includes tofu, miso soup, or tempeh. Soybeans have the highest protein content in the legume family, but unfermented, they also contain enzyme inhibitors that can block the absorption of important nutrients.

One of the most versatile and easy-to-use soy foods in tofu. I know, tofu has gotten a bad rap. But that's only because most people don't know how to prepare it. Tofu is soybean curd. Dried soybeans are soaked in water and then crushed and boiled. The remaining soy milk is separated from the pulp, and a curdling agent is added to separate out the curds. The fresh, warm curds are poured into square molds where, as they cool, they become firm.

The final product is a mild-tasting, white, cheese-like cake that is stored in cool water to keep it fresh. Tofu is high in protein, cholesterol-free, and low in sodium. Although soybeans are higher in fat than most legumes, they contain virtually no saturated fat and are high in linoleic acid, an important essential fatty acid.

Tofu varies in texture and firmness. Firm and extra firm tofu is dense and holds its shape when you cook it. It's higher in protein and fat than the other forms. Silken tofu is softer, with a creamier consistency and works well for pureed, blended or scrambled tofu.

Tofu is stored in cool water to keep it fresh. If you use part of a package of tofu, cover the remainder with water and store it in the refrigerator.

Because tofu is very mild and soaks up any flavor you add to it, it has a virtually unlimited number of uses. It can substitute for meat in chili, for cheese in lasagna or it can even be barbecued on a grill with barbecue sauce. I have a friend who makes scrambled tofu instead of scrambled eggs for breakfast, and then adds ketchup. Now there's an interesting combination of Asian and American tastes! The Japanese like to eat tofu in miso soup with scallions and mushrooms (miso is a fermented soybean paste that is added to hot water to make a soup). I especially like tofu added to stir-fried veggies. The key to learning to love tofu is to begin by adding it to dishes you already love: spaghetti and other Italian dishes, casseroles, soups and stews, for example.

Adzuki or Aduki Beans are small red beans originally from Asia. They are high in nutrients, have a nice sweet flavor, a soft texture, and cook faster than most beans because they're small. They combine very nicely with basmati rice, an aromatic rice with a distinctive flavor and mix well with other grains and dishes such as soups and casseroles. Cooking ratio is 2 to 3 cups water to 1 cup beans, simmer for 1½ hours, less if soaked.

Black Beans or Black Turtle Beans are what you often find in Mexican food. They are a more robust bean with an earthy flavor. They tend to retain more of their shape and texture after cooking than most beans and do well with strong seasonings such as garlic and cumin. Cooking ratio is 2 to 3 cups water to 1 cup beans, simmer for 2½ hours, less if soaked.

Lentils are much smaller and flatter than most beans and are widely used in the Middle East, where there are dozens of varieties. They cook quickly and have their own unique flavor. They mix well in casseroles, soups and salads. Cooking ratio is 2 to 4 cups water to 1 cup beans, simmer for 1 hour, less if soaked.

Black Bean Soup

This recipe serves four.

In wintertime, there's nothing more warming and nutritious than black bean soup. Here's my favorite recipe. You can vary the vegetables and spices to suit your personal tastes.

2 cups dried black beans

6 cups water

2 tbs. unrefined olive oil

½ to 1 medium onion, diced

3 cloves garlic, crushed

1 large carrot, chopped

2 stalks celery, chopped

Juice of ½ a lemon or 1 cup orange juice

1 tsp. ground coriander

1½ tsp. ground cumin

A dash of cayenne

1 bay leaf

½ tsp. sea salt

Soak the beans overnight and then discard the soaking water. Bring water and beans to a boil and let simmer for 1 hour.

Sauté the onion, garlic, carrot, coriander, cumin, cayenne and salt.

When the beans have cooked for one hour, add the sautéed vegetables and spices.

Add the bay leaf and lemon juice and continue cooking until the beans are tender.

A variation of this is to puree the beans in a blender after they have cooked for an hour, and then add the vegetables. I like to add fresh cilantro and a dollop of nonfat plain yogurt to my black bean soup. Some people like to add salsa.

Six Good Reasons to Eat Yogurt

Dairy products are a good source of protein, but some are better foods than others, and yogurt is one of my favorite healthy foods. I would like to see most everyone eating yogurt containing "live cultures" at least a few times a week. Why should you eat yogurt? I can think of six good reasons:

1. Yogurt is a great source of calcium. Calcium is important for strong bones and teeth, calming the nerves, and necessary for every beat of your heart. Yogurt contains fermented cultures containing the "good" bacteria found in your digestive system. These bacteria are essential to proper digestion, and aid the body in absorbing calcium.

2. Yogurt can help reduce cholesterol. Many recent studies indicate that the fermented cultures in yogurt help lower cholesterol.

3. Yogurt can help your immune system do its job. It has been a folk remedy for colds, diarrhea and fighting infections for centuries, and now scientific research is validating this. There is even some evidence that eating yogurt daily can help reduce hay fever symptoms.

4. Yogurt can help fight cancer. All that and this too? You bet! Scientists don't understand exactly why, but research indicates that yogurt seems to block the development of cancers. There's something about those "good" bacteria that inspires the immune system to destroy tumor cells.

5. Yogurt can reduce lactose intolerance. Lactose is milk sugar that many people (some say as much as 70 percent of the adult population) have trouble digesting. Lactose intolerance can cause chronic gas, intestinal cramps and allergy symptoms. However, lactose-intolerant people who eat yogurt regularly seem to develop a much greater ability to digest lactose.

6. Yogurt can help reduce or eliminate ulcers. About 40 years ago, scientists discovered that too much of a specific bacteria in the stomach causes ulcers. Unfortunately this research was ignored until recently when it was "rediscovered," and in spite of tremendous resistance from the medical and pharmaceutical community it is now official: the friendly bacteria in yogurt helps destroy the bacteria that cause ulcers and many other digestive difficulties.

Antibiotics kill bacteria in the digestive system, including the "good" bacteria. If you take antibiotics, please be sure to follow them up with a half cup of yogurt twice daily for at least two weeks. If you can't tolerate yogurt for some reason you can buy acidophilus in capsules at your local health food store.

Yogurt Tips. I strongly recommend that you buy plain yogurt, free of sweeteners (natural or artificial), artificial colors and preservatives. You can sweeten or flavor it yourself with honey, maple syrup (a little of these sweeteners goes a long way, or fruit, or find a brand that is fruit-sweetened only. Adding a drop of vanilla can also make plain yogurt more palatable. Kids often love yogurt with a crunchy cereal such as granola sprinkled on it. (Please pass on the yogurt that comes with toppings. They tend to be high in fat and sugar.)

CHAPTER 7

Dissecting the Food
We All Hate to Love

FAT CAN
BE YOUR
FRIEND

IT WOULD BE NO EXAGGERATION TO SAY that over the past few years, hundreds of people have written me to tell me that they're eating almost no fat and getting plenty of exercise, yet they are constantly fatigued and continue to gain weight. In general, women who don't eat fat get hormonal imbalances, and men who don't eat fat tend to get depressed. In this chapter I'm going to explain why fat is an essential part of your diet, and how to be smart about which fats you eat.

Fat is the third essential source for fuel in your diet, yet unfortunately it also describes unwanted excess. But not all fats automatically make you fat. Certain types of fat are actually necessary for sustaining the body's life support systems. What's more, they can also aid in increasing insulin sensitivity and weight loss.

Fats form much of the structure of the body, from cell membranes to a biological cushion that protects and insulates. In foods, fats add flavor and a smooth, pleasing texture. Because they take longer to digest, certain fats continue to let us feel full even after the proteins and carbohydrates have been emptied from the stomach.

Fats are necessary for the transport and absorption of the fat-soluble vitamins A, D, E, and K, and they are building blocks for the sex hormones, as well as those that regulate the metabolism of food and energy.

FAT BASICS

Fats can be derived from animals or plants, and in their natural form are saturated, monounsaturated, or unsaturated. In general, saturated fats, including animal fats, butter, and coconut oil are solid at room temperature.

Monounsaturated fats (olive and canola oil) are liquid at room temperature and solid or semisolid under refrigeration. Polyunsaturated fats (corn and sunflower oils), are always liquid. Partially hydrogenated oils are man-made, and have hydrogen added in the process called hydrogenation, as in the making of margarine. These man-made oils are also called trans-fatty acids, and you should strictly avoid them—I'll explain why shortly.

There are some fatty acids that are called "essential," and for good reasons. Essential fatty acids (EFAs) ensure proper growth, muscle strength, and brain functions and support the adrenal and thyroid glands that regulate metabolism and energy production. They keep your skin and other tissues healthy and make your hair strong and shiny. There are a total of eight essential fatty acids, which generally fall into two classes—omega-6 and omega-3. Omega 6 fatty acids are found mainly in vegetables oils, and omega 3 fatty acids are found mainly in nuts, seeds, and fish. I will discuss these at length, but first, let's look at the historical sources for fat.

COMING FULL CIRCLE WITH FATS

It is estimated that our Paleolithic ancestors derived 20 to 25 percent of their diet from fat, mainly in the form of muscle and organ meats, but also from nuts, seeds, and plants. With the advent of domesticated animals and agriculture 10,000 years ago, people began to get some of their fat from dairy products, but they still extracted many of their oils from fish, fish liver, olives, animal fats, peanuts, coconuts, palms, and sesame seeds.

When industrialization allowed us to use high pressure and temperatures to cheaply extract oils from corn, soy, and safflower, the omega-6 fatty acids began to overshadow the omega-3 fatty acids in our diet, thus setting the stage for insulin resistance syndrome. The omega-6 oils are unsaturated and easily become rancid, so we learned to artificially saturate liquid vegetable oil with hydrogen to form solid fats (trans-fatty acids, also called hydrogenated oils) which could sit on store shelves for weeks and even months without spoiling. In the 1930s, we began using toxic solvents to squeeze even more oil out of the plants. These processes made vegetable oil widely available, but destroyed the protective antioxidants in the oils, thus raising our cholesterol levels and putting us at risk for heart disease and diabetes.

However, thanks to aggressive marketing and advertising campaigns on the part of the vegetable oil industry, and manipulation of government regulatory agencies, the deleterious effects of trans-fatty acids were swept under the rug for decades, and we were told that they were good for us. Health organizations, such as the American Heart Association, blamed saturated fat for the proliferation of heart disease, and launched an aggressive three-decade campaign against cholesterol that advocated the use of omega-6-rich vegetable oils and corn-oil margarines.

Researchers today are beginning to understand that in an effort to combat excess fat, soaring cholesterol and triglyceride levels, heart disease, and diabetes, we only made the problem worse.

THE YIN AND YANG OF ESSENTIAL FATTY ACIDS

A balanced diet contains the unsaturated essential fatty acids (EFAs), omega-6 and omega-3, or linoleic acid and alpha-linolenic acid, respectively. Many of the fatty acids we need to support the normal structure and function of cells can be made from these two fats. Linoleic acid is commonly found in most food groups. Alpha-linolenic acid is an even more unsaturated fat belonging to the omega-3 family found in flaxseed oil, and in smaller amounts in canola oil, soybeans, walnuts, and dark green vegetables. (Because canola and soy oils are so high in omega-6 fats, they aren't good oils to consume to get omega-3 oils.) Alpha-linolenic acid is a precursor to two important oils called eicosapentaenoic acid (EPA) and docosahexaenoic acid (DHA). Fish is a great source of these oils, and to a lesser degree eggs are too.

All in all, it is unhealthy for dietary fats to be skewed one way or another. The ratio of omega-6 oils to omega-3 oils should be about two to one or even three to one, but in our modern diet with its refined foods, it tends to be much higher than that. In the process of replacing saturated fats (from meat and eggs) with vegetable oils (such as soy, corn, and safflower oils), the omega-3 fats (found in fish) have virtually been forced out of the modern diet. People today consume 20 to 30 times more omega-6 than omega-3 fats.

An imbalance of the omega-6 and omega-3 predisposes us to chronic diseases by making us more susceptible to insulin resistance and high triglycerides, both risk factors for heart disease. A half-dozen studies have linked low levels of omega-3 fatty acids in the blood with depression, schizophrenia, attention deficit disorder, and aggressiveness. The risk of developing these problems is exaggerated even more when we eat the partially hydrogenated oils found in margarine and many other processed food products, because they interfere with the proper storage and metabolism of the EFAs.

Of particular importance to those who are obese and suffering from insulin resistance is that the body needs the omega-3 fatty acids to produce flexible cell membranes, which contain numerous insulin receptors that should be receptive and responsive to insulin. Without sufficient omega-3 fatty acids (especially one particular type, called DHA found in fish oils), the membranes are not as flexible, and insulin resistance can develop. Adding omega-3 oils to the diet can reverse insulin resistance.

In one study, nine obese patients with type 2 diabetes were treated with a diet enriched in omega-3 and monounsaturated fats, while eight other obese patients with type 2 diabetes were placed on a low-fat, high-carbohydrate diet. Both groups lost weight at about the same rate, but the group that ate a greater amount of monounsaturated fat and omega-3 fatty acids, had a greater decrease in total cholesterol and triglycerides. Omega-3 fatty acids protect against cardiovascular disease and stroke by reducing platelet aggregation (the tendency of blood clots to form).

A high ratio of omega-6 to omega-3 fatty acids may promote obesity, as well. One study on mice compared the effects of diets rich in omega-6 soybean oil to diets rich in omega-3 fish oils. The mice on soybean oil got fatter than those on the fish oil. The mice on fish oil actually became leaner. This same phenomenon is just starting to be seen in research with humans. One study found that people whose muscle cells contain low levels of omega-3 fatty acids and high levels of omega-6 fatty acids are more likely to be insulin resistant and obese.

Here's how to strike a balance between omega-6 and omega-3 fats in the diet:

- First, since omega-6 oils are so prevalent in American diets, cut back on all vegetable oils except extra-virgin olive oil. Avoid corn, soybean, safflower, sunflower, and cottonseed oil, all high in omega-6 fatty acids. These are found in nearly all processed foods, so read food labels.
- Replace omega-6 oils with unrefined or cold-pressed extra-virgin olive oil, which is a monounsaturated fat, as your primary oil in salads and cooking. Olive oil is low in omega-6 fatty acids and rich in omega-9 monounsaturated fatty acids, which do not compete with omega-3 fatty acids in the body.
- The easiest way to improve your omega-3 fatty acid intake is to eat cold-water fish, such as salmon, trout, tuna, sardines, herring, and anchovies two to three times a week. Fish is rich

in "preformed" DHA and eicosapentaenoic acid (EPA), so eating
these fish even once a week reduces your risk of heart attack.
An alternative to eating fish is to take 1 to 3 grams of fish oil
in capsule form daily. Make sure the oil contains vitamin E to
prevent rancidity, and is purified to remove toxins.

- Add chopped walnuts, high in omega-3, on top of cereals or
  salads, or in baked goods, or eat a few walnuts as snacks.
- Try to find omega-3 enriched eggs and meats. A number of egg
  producers feed their animals a mash enriched with fish meal or
  flaxseeds and, sometimes, vitamin E.
- Search out meat and milk products from free-range animals that
  eat omega-3-rich grass rather than omega-6-rich grains.
- Try game meat such as venison, buffalo, or game birds, which
  more closely resemble the fatty-acid ratios of Paleolithic meats.
- Dark-green leafy vegetables, including romaine lettuce, mixed
  greens, arugula, kale, collards, mustard greens, and Swiss chard,
  are good sources of omega-3 fatty acids.
- Add foods that contain monounsaturated fats to your diet,
  including almonds, pistachios, pecans, hazelnuts, cashews,
  macadamia nuts, and avocados. Monounsaturated fats increase
  levels of good HDL cholesterol and inhibit the oxidation of
  the bad LDL cholesterol. Substituting monounsaturated fats
  for carbohydrates also improves insulin sensitivity. Although
  peanut oil is a monounsaturated fat and is fairly stable, peanuts
  are highly susceptible to a type of fungus containing poisonous
  aflatoxin. It also tends to be a crop heavily sprayed with pesticides
  and fungicides. I don't recommend peanut oil unless it's organic
  and from a highly reputable source.

AVOID TRANS-FATTY ACIDS

Some processed foods and baked goods contain trans-fatty acids, also
called partially hydrogenated oils. This is a good reason to avoid all of these
types of foods, because evidence is growing that these man-made "fake fats"
may be at the root of our ever-growing rate of heart disease and cancer.

Trans-fatty acids promote insulin resistance and a variety of health problems in the body because they are shaped differently than the polyunsaturated fatty acids from which they are made. They act like misfits by crowding

out essential fats from the cell membranes and interfering with the conversion of shorter-chain fatty acids into longer ones. Fewer long-chain fatty acids are thus incorporated into cell membranes, which reduces the number of insulin receptors on their surface, and makes them less fluid and sensitive to insulin.

In one study, women who ate margarine four or more times per week had high triglycerides, low HDL cholesterol, and high total cholesterol, three of the four symptoms of insulin resistance syndrome. Furthermore, animal experiments have found that trans-fatty acids promote obesity by increasing the size of fat cells. Large fat cells have fewer insulin receptors and store more fat than normal fat cells.

To prevent insulin resistance and its serious complications, you can significantly reduce your intake of trans-fatty acids by avoiding fried foods, margarine, vegetable shortening, many microwavable and TV dinners, crackers, cookies, cakes, and other convenience foods.

IS SATURATED FAT BAD FOR ME?

This is going to surprise you, but the answer is no! Saturated fat is not bad for you. Saturated fats are easy to digest and you burn them up quickly and efficiently. Saturated fats are needed by the body to convert some of the EFAs into other important types of important fatty acids within the body. They are essential for supporting your body's ability to fight harmful bacteria and viruses, and are also essential in protecting you from cancer.

Too much saturated fat is unhealthy. In the 1950s Americans got into the habit of eating large amounts of saturated fat morning, noon and night, and that's not healthy.

Saturated fat is found in the highest concentrations in red meat, butter, coconut oil, and other tropical oils. It is also found in smaller concentrations (6 to 20 percent) in all other oils. The total amount of saturated fat in your diet can range from as low as 5 percent of your total calories, up to about 10 percent of your total calories, or half of your total fat intake. I'm not going to give you an exact amount of saturated fat to eat, because that can vary from person to person. Some people thrive on saturated fat, while others do best on very small amounts. Again, you need to experiment to find out what works best for you.

BUT DON'T STUDIES LINK SATURATED FAT TO HEART ATTACKS?

Keep in mind that it's the excess of saturated fat that causes problems. Most heart disease studies involving saturated fats have missed some key factors. First, the studies dealing with tropical oil consumption (saturated fat such as coconut oil or palm oil) involved refined oils. Many populations around the world consume unrefined tropical oils as a major part of their diet, and they are quite healthy and free of heart disease.

Another error in these studies is not comparing total fat intake to the saturated fat eaten. According to population studies, people who eat too much saturated fat tend to lead less healthy lives in general. They don't exercise much; they eat too much refined sugar; and they don't get enough fiber, fresh fruits, or vegetables. All of these factors weigh heavily in heart disease.

Third, the amount of trans-fatty acids eaten was a factor left out of these studies, and now we know that it is most likely these fats that are causing the heart disease, not the saturated fats.

Eating saturated fat does not raise cholesterol levels except in a very small percentage of the population. This is a mistaken notion promoted by the vegetable oil industry. Your body manufactures about 75 percent of its cholesterol, and the rest is supplied from your diet. Any excess cholesterol is simply excreted. Cholesterol is essential for proper brain function, and it is a precursor to all of your steroid hormones (cortisones, progesterone, estrogen, testosterone, etc.).

High cholesterol is a symptom of heart disease, not a disease in and of itself. Heart disease patients often have higher cholesterol levels than patients who don't have heart disease, but fully one third of people who have a heart attack have none of the conventional medical risk factors, and many people with high cholesterol never have heart disease. The issue with cholesterol is oxidation: It is oxidized LDL cholesterol that promotes damage to the arteries and clogs them with plaques. Maintaining good antioxidant levels is more important than how much cholesterol you eat, as is maintaining good levels of HDL cholesterol, which aids in its removal from the bloodstream.

It would be a mistake to assume that by simply lowering your cholesterol levels with drugs you can prevent heart disease. You need to address the underlying factors that caused the rise in the first place. Taking steps to control your insulin and blood sugar will improve your cholesterol profile (lowering LDL and raising your HDL), and that will certainly help keep your heart healthy.

Carbohydrates, protein, and fat form the major acts of the three-ring circus that is necessary to run the body. But what about all the side shows of nutrition? Vitamins and minerals, the micronutrients, perform specific functions that are essential to insulin and glucose control, circulation, absorption, and a host of other balancing acts. Furthermore, nature has provided us with miraculous plants that can help us to balance our blood sugar when we need a little extra help. In the following chapters, I'll explore these nutritional tools in detail.

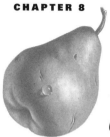

CHAPTER 8

The Asian Secret to Blood Sugar Balance and Weight Loss

BANABA: THE DIVINE FLOWER

PETER HAD JUST SUFFERED FROM A mild heart attack, and his doctor told him that if he didn't lose weight his next one could be more serious. He was highly motivated to change his diet and get more exercise, but just couldn't seem to get past the cravings for carbohydrates. He would find himself in the kitchen in the middle of the afternoon getting corn chips, and at the junk food drive-up window getting a large order of fries to eat on the way home.

Peter is not at all unusual—once you develop a sugar and carbohydrate habit it can be very difficult to get control of your cravings for those foods and stabilize your blood sugar. This is why it can be useful to use natural supplements such as banaba to help balance insulin levels. Combined with the nutrients I'll tell you about in the following chapter, you have powerful weapons in the battle of the bulge.

Modern help for people suffering from obesity and high blood sugar disorders comes from an ancient source. Banaba is a traditional herbal medicine for hyperglycemia and diabetes that has been used for centuries in Southeast Asia. Herbal lore from the Philippines, Thailand, Indonesia, Malaysia, South China, India, and Australia all refers to the benefits of banaba.

The name "banaba" comes from the Tagalog language of the Philippines. Banaba, or *Lagerstroemia speciosa*, is a variety of the Crape Myrtle tree. It is a beautiful hardwood shade tree growing up to 60 feet high with an outward canopy of 40 to 60 feet. An abundance of large, three-inch wide, sprays of flowers bloom during the summer. The flowers have a wide variety of colors.

Because of its lovely appearance, banaba has a variety of common names such as "Divine Flower" and the "Rose of India." Its leaves are approximately 12 inches long, oblong, leathery, and dark green in color, turning an attractive red before falling in winter. The tree grows wild in the Philippines.

In the United States banaba is grown as a decorative plant on highways, and in residential areas as a shade tree. It is one of the few deciduous trees which grow in tropical or sub-tropical areas of the country such as Hawaii, Florida, and in other Southeastern states where it is called "Queen's Crape Myrtle."

The leaves and flowers of the banaba tree can be used as a tea. Diabetic patients in the Philippines drink the tea as a tonic. It is caffeine-free, safe for the liver, and has no known negative side effects for people with high blood sugar. In addition to banaba's benefits for blood sugar problems, it can also be helpful for other diseases such as obesity, high blood pressure, kidney problems, ulcers, abdominal pain and wound healing. The tea has diuretic properties, meaning it helps the body to excrete excess fluids, which can be useful for people suffering from water retention. Banaba also acts as an antioxidant, helping to scavenge free radicals and preventing cell membrane lipid peroxidation.

Banaba came into the spotlight of modern medicine and research in the early 1990s when a Japanese businessman involved in the confectioners' industry, on vacation in the Philippines, was introduced to a banaba plant growing in a local garden. He took a sample back with him to Japan and, due to his interest, research on its properties began.

In the United Sates there are an estimated 22.4 million people with type 2 diabetes, and it is estimated that worldwide there are 110 million diabetics. According to the World Health Organization (WHO), the next century will probably see the number of diabetics worldwide rise to 200 million in both developed and third world countries. This is because Western industrialized countries are importing their poor dietary habits of eating too much sugar and over-refined carbohydrates and not enough fresh vegetables and fruits, to the rest of the world.

The magnitude of this worldwide high blood sugar problem has spurred an interest in continuing research into solutions that go beyond dietary changes.

THE INNER MAGIC OF BANABA

What is it that makes banaba so useful for high blood sugar conditions? Powder from the banaba leaf contains a substance called corosolic acid, which has been shown to have some of insulin's properties in the body. Corosolic acid is what is known as a glucose transport activator. Discovered by Professor Kazuo Yamazaki of the Medical Department of Hiroshima University, it has the ability to help to transport excess sugar from the bloodstream directly across cell membranes into the cells. When excess sugar remains in the blood, it can be damaging to other parts of the body such as the arteries, and the cells are starved for fuel.

Banaba is a breakthrough in the world of treatment for diabetes because, except for insulin itself, virtually no other substance has the ability to regulate the amount of sugar in the bloodstream. Corosolic acid is therefore known as an insulin-like plant extract or phtyo-insulin.

RESEARCH ON BANABA LOOKS GOOD

In one study in Japan at the Tokyo Jikeikai Medical School, 24 people with mild type 2 diabetes took part in a crossover, double-blind, placebo-controlled four-week study. The participants were given oral doses of either a standardized corosolic acid tablet or a placebo, three times daily following meals. The results showed that corosolic acid is effective in lowering blood glucose levels. The results continued for the participants for a few days following the study.

Clinical studies with humans in the U.S. have also shown promising results. A series of studies conducted by Dr. William Judy at the Southeastern Institute of Biomedical Research in Bradenton, Florida, focused on the ability of corolic acid to lower blood sugar, and on how this effect is related to different dosages.

One of these studies was a series of randomized, double-blind crossover studies with twelve diabetic subjects for 22 weeks. This group of people also suffered from type 2 diabetes. The participants initially took doses of 16, 32, and 48 mg of the banaba extract per day for two weeks. The corosolic acid was given in the form of an oil-based gelatin capsule. With the 16 mg dose, blood sugar levels dropped 4.9 percent. At the 32 mg dose, levels dropped 10.7 percent, and at 48 mg the drop was 31.9 percent, compared to the placebo.

Corosolic acid also facilitates a sharper decline of glucose levels directly after meals. Typically blood sugar levels will spike for the diabetic after a meal whereas a person with normal blood sugar won't experience this. Diabetics using banaba or corosolic acid supplementation also report experiencing less thirst and urination, again common symptoms of diabetes.

Another piece of good news about banaba's effect on blood sugar is that it tends to create gradual weight loss caused by the reduction in fat storage, and this is much better for the body than rapid weight loss. Researchers believe that the weight loss is caused by the way that blood sugar is metabolized in the presence of banaba. Insulin converts excess blood sugar into fat. Banaba, in contrast, allows excess sugar to be more effectively burned as energy by the cells. In other words, the body goes into fat *burning* rather than fat storage mode. This result occurred in the research using both animal and human participants. In one study with humans, subjects lost an average of 3.2 pounds after 45 days without any changes to the diet. Participants also reported that their appetite was somewhat reduced, which may be due to the more efficient use of blood sugars for energy.

Another difference between banaba and insulin is that banaba can be taken orally to produce a drop in blood sugar, whereas insulin has to be injected to produce the same effect. In addition, dosages of insulin must be monitored for safety, while banaba has no known adverse side effects. It can be taken orally, as tea, in capsule or tablet form.

While banaba can be useful for people suffering from high blood sugar and diabetes, it may not be suitable in higher doses for people with normal blood sugar. Interestingly, when a diabetic uses banaba their blood sugar tends to normalize, and will not tend to fall below normal levels. However, there is some indication that in people with normal blood sugar levels higher doses of banaba may cause blood sugar to drop too much. Thus, if you have a tendency towards hypoglycemia (low blood sugar), use banaba with caution at first to see if it works for you.

In smaller doses, banaba can be very useful even if you have normal blood sugar, if it's taken after a meal, and as part of a low-sugar low-carbohydrate diet, because it encourages blood sugar stability after a meal. It can be especially useful when combined with other natural blood sugar-lowering remedies such as vanadium and chromium.

WHERE TO FIND BANABA

I chew a supplement that contains the banaba extract, chromium, hoodia, gymnema sylvestre and citrus aurantium that all work together to curb the desire for processed carbohydrates and sugar. I chew one or two tablets at the beginning of each meal, twice daily.

You can find banaba at your local health food store or online, often in a formula for blood sugar control.

CHAPTER 9

Herbal Secrets and Nutritional Supplements

NATURAL REMEDIES FOR BLOOD SUGAR BALANCE

THE INDUSTRIAL REVOLUTION THAT ALLOWED US to mechanize food preparation, increase agricultural production, and work more efficiently also sapped us of the micronutrients we need to keep our bodies humming as well as our machinery. Mounting evidence shows that obesity, insulin resistance, and type 2 diabetes not only develop from a misguided diet and a sedentary lifestyle, but also may be tied to deficiencies of certain vitamins and minerals. Just as we can reverse obesity and insulin resistance with diet, we can greatly expedite the healing process with nutritional and natural supplements.

Keep in mind that these supplements will affect your blood sugar, so if you have diagnosed diabetes, don't take them without closely monitoring your glucose until you find out how they affect your blood sugar balance. You should be able to find all of these supplements at your health food store and the health food sections in many grocery stores. If you have unstable blood sugar or are diabetic, please work in partnership with a qualified health care professional who can help you monitor your health. I devoted a full chapter to banaba because I'm convinced that it's a breakthrough in natural remedies for balancing blood sugar, but even banaba works best in combination with these other herbs, vitamins, minerals, and other supplements.

BLOOD SUGAR-BALANCING HERBS

Chinese and **Siberian ginseng root (*Panax ginseng* and *Eletherococcus senticosus)*** have been used in Asia for centuries, and can reduce fasting blood glucose and stimulate metabolism for added energy. Take ginseng with a 5 to 7 percent ginsenoside content.

Gymenma sylvestre is an Ayurvedic herb from India that lowers blood sugar. There is also some evidence that 400 mg of gymenma sylvestre a day actually reverses damage to certain cells in the pancreas that can be destroyed by diabetes. You can find it at your health food store, but be sure to tell your healthcare provider that you are taking this herb because if you are taking diabetes drugs, they may need to be adjusted.

Gugulipid, the active component in gugul, is a plant used in East Indian Ayurvedic medicine to treat obesity. Published studies have shown that gugulipid significantly reduces cholesterol with results comparable to prescription anti-cholesterol drugs, but without the side effects. It also increases HDL levels. Take one to three 500 mg tablets daily with water.

Bitter melon *(Momordica charantia)* is a tropical fruit tested extensively in clinical trials and proven effective in balancing blood sugar.

Juniper berry, a major component of many indigenous diets, is useful for detoxifying and controlling blood sugar.

Burdock root *(Arctium lappa)* is high in *inulin,* a compound that acts like insulin.

Griffonia simplicifolia seed assists in appetite control, and *Phaseolus vulgaris* seed acts as an inhibitor to amylase, the enzyme which helps break down starches into sugar.

Licorice root *(Glycyrrhiza glabra)*, ginger root *(Zingiber officinales)*, and astragalus root *(Astragalus membranaceus)* support the adrenal glands, which can be put under stress on a low-carbohydrate diet when there is increased fat-burning activity.

FAT-BURNING SUPPLEMENTS

The best way to shift your metabolism into a higher gear and lose weight is to exercise. If you're working to change to a healthier lifestyle and want to give yourself a little extra boost, here are some fat-burning supplements that can help change your metabolism. However, I want to emphasize that these are not magic pills that will work without exercise and good nutrition, and they are only meant to be used for a couple of weeks to a few months, to get you going.

Garcinia Cambogia The fruit of the plant *Garcinia cambogia* is commonly used in Asia as a food, spice, or condiment, where it is said to enhance digestion and make food seem more filling. Garcinia is a lipogenesis inhibitor, meaning it interferes with the body's ability to convert and store fats from carbohydrates and proteins. Studies done on rats by the pharmaceutical company Hoffman-La Roche have shown that a substance in garcinia called hydroxycitrate HCA suppresses appetite, reduces the body's ability to use fatty acids, and reduces the conversion of carbohydrates to fat. Because it is eaten in Asia as a food, I feel it is safe to use to assist with weight loss and change in metabolism, for a limited amount of time.

Look for a garcinia supplement that guarantees a 50 percent HCA content. Follow the directions on the container. Most of the supplements recommend 1,500 to 3,000 mg daily in divided doses. It's best to take garcinia half an hour before meals, as it suppresses appetite.

You should know that all of the studies done with garcinia on humans have combined it with other weight-loss supplements, such as chromium glycinate, so there is some controversy as to whether garcinia works as effectively by itself.

Gamma-linolenic Acid (GLA) Much attention has been given recently to the wonders of aspirin. While aspirin does enhance the process of thermogenesis, or the burning of fats, its side effects make it not worth the risk except in very small amounts. However, you can give yourself the same benefits as aspirin by making sure your gamma-linolenic acid (GLA) levels are high. GLA is an omega-6 fatty acid normally made in the body from the essential fatty acid linoleic acid.

GLA plays an essential role in the formation of "good" prostaglandins in the body, which are hormone-like substances that, among other things such as inhibiting inflammation, help the body burn fat more easily.

The best way to insure that your GLA levels stay high and in balance with the other fatty acids is to avoid those things that deplete GLA. The biggest offenders are the trans-fatty acids found in hydrogenated oils. These "fake" oils rob the body of GLA. The next biggest offenders are processed foods which are depleted of GLA. Whole grains, and particularly oatmeal, as well as many nuts and seeds, contain small amounts of GLA. Taking too much alpha-linolenic acid, the omega-3 fatty acid found in flax seed oil, is another way to suppress GLA production. Flax seed oil is something of a nutritional fad right now, but I don't recommend you take large amounts of it long term as it is a highly unstable unsaturated oil that can do just as much harm as good if it's rancid or taken in excess.

You can also take GLA in the form of a supplement of evening primrose oil or borage oil. Follow the directions on the container.

ESSENTIAL MINERALS FOR INSULIN AND BLOOD SUGAR CONTROL

Chromium is a centerpiece supplement for blood sugar control, and it follows that the lack of this mineral may be one of the root causes of insulin resistance and diabetes. An estimated 90 million people in the U.S. are actually deficient in chromium and high fructose corn syrup may be one of the reasons: As our consumption of this syrup has increased 250 percent in the past 15 years, during the same period, our rate of diabetes has increased approximately 45 percent. Fructose consumption causes a drop in chromium, raises LDL "bad" cholesterol and triglycerides, and impairs immune system function, according to studies done at the Agriculture Department's Human Nutrition Resource Center.

Chromium helps the body break down carbohydrates. It occurs naturally in root vegetables such as carrots and potatoes, in whole grains, and in some beers and wines. Chromium can actually make you gain weight if you continue on a diet dominated by refined carbohydrates and sugar, because it does such a fantastic job in helping your body stuff sugar into cells.

But on the correct diet, in combination with other supplements described in this chapter, and exercise, chromium is a useful aid in weight reduction. Chromium helps control sugar cravings, which in turn keeps you from grabbing high-calorie snacks and fast food meals. It can increase total lean body mass, which in turn increases metabolism. Chromium has been found to have beneficial effects on blood fats, such as decreasing LDL cholesterol and triglycerides and increasing HDL cholesterol, which makes it an excellent supplement for combating the other symptoms of insulin resistance syndrome.

In people with mild insulin resistance, 200 mcg per day should be enough to help improve insulin levels. Chromium does affect your blood sugar, so if you are on medication for controlling your glucose, it's important to closely monitor your blood sugar.

If you treat yourself to an occasional dessert, you can take 200 mg of chromium to counteract the siege of glucose and insulin about two hours after taking it. Otherwise, that piece of chocolate cake will likely effect your glucose for six to eight hours, making you feel miserable. If you know you are going to do this, make sure you don't eat other carbohydrates, but do try to eat enough protein and fish or olive oil during that same sitting to help protect you from overdosing on glucose.

Chromium glycinate is the best-absorbed form of this mineral.

Zinc plays a critical role in glucose regulation, but because of our tendency to choose processed foods and avoid zinc-rich foods, most Americans are deficient in it. Zinc deficiencies put people at greater risk for glucose intolerance, diabetes, coronary artery disease, and obesity. When there is not enough zinc, the pancreas makes inadequate amounts of insulin to counter high glucose levels. The insulin that is released doesn't work as effectively. Zinc allows the pancreas to work more effectively to produce more insulin and helps maintain insulin sensitivity. Zinc also effects blood levels of leptin, a hormone that influences appetite, energy, and body composition. If zinc is low in the body, you never feel full and tend to overindulge on poor quality carbohydrates.

Optimal amounts of zinc vary widely among individuals, but 30 mg is a good dose for men, and 15 mg daily for women.

Copper and zinc are commonly recommended in combination, but they can adversely effect one another. Zinc can cause copper deficiency, which can effect HDL and LDL cholesterol ratios in the wrong way. Conversely, when zinc levels are low in the body, copper levels tend to build up, and high levels of copper can cause heart disease and obesity, as well as retinopathy, hypertension, and microvascular complications. Diabetics and people suffering from insulin resistance syndrome usually have low levels of zinc and excessive levels of copper. If you have either condition, avoid taking copper supplements. Diabetics can still get all the copper they need from nuts and seeds.

Iron, like copper, can adversely affect cholesterol levels. In excess, iron can create too much oxidation in the body. Do not take supplements containing iron unless you've been diagnosed with a deficiency. Try to avoid iron-fortified foods like enriched white flour and white rice (the very carbohydrates that help to cause diabetes!). You can still get all the iron you need from meat, eggs, poultry, and spinach. (Pregnant or lactating women, particularly those who have gestational diabetes, should consult a nutritionally oriented health care provider.)

Magnesium is yet another mineral found to be deficient in type 2 diabetics. Like zinc, it is necessary for the production and release of insulin, and is required by the cells for maintaining insulin sensitivity. Without adequate magnesium levels in the body, insulin is less able to move glucose from the blood into the cells. Magnesium helps to prevent and reverse high blood pressure and keeps blood platelets from clumping together to form blood clots, thereby preventing complications of insulin resistance that lead to heart disease and stroke.

Magnesium can be depleted by stress, excessive alcohol, sugar, diabetes, kidney disease, chronic diarrhea, not enough protein in the diet, too much protein in the diet, and thyroid disorders. Alcoholics are at a much greater risk for heart disease. Many researchers believe the increased risk is caused by the depletion effect excess alcohol has on magnesium.

Drugs that can deplete magnesium include corticosteroids (Prednisone), loop and thiazide diuretics used to lower blood pressure, aminoglycosides (antibiotics such as streptomycin, gentamicin, and amikacin), and cisplatin (a chemotherapy drug).

Good food sources of magnesium include whole grains (especially oats, brown rice, millet, buckwheat, and wheat), legumes (lentils, split peas, and beans), bran, almonds, peanuts, and broccoli. Chocolate contains large amounts of magnesium, and a craving for chocolate may be an indicator of a magnesium deficiency.

Magnesium by itself can cause diarrhea, so unless you are constipated, be sure to take it in a multivitamin, in combination with calcium, or in the form of magnesium glycinate, magnesium citrate, or magnesium aspartate.

I recommend that you take 300 to 400 mg of magnesium daily as a supplement. Studies show that vegetarians tend to have very good magnesium levels—yet another good reason to eat lots of whole grains, fresh fruits, and vegetables.

Vanadium, a trace mineral taken in the form of vanadyl sulfate, works by mimicking insulin, thereby helping cells to absorb sugar more effectively and lowering cholesterol and triglyceride levels. It is present in the earth's crust and is, therefore, present in any food that contains earth salts, like vegetables and meat.

Long-term high doses of vanadium are not recommended, but you can use it to help stabilize your blood sugar for a period. You can start with 6 mg daily and work your way up to 100 mg per day, under the supervision of a health care professional if you are diabetic. Once you begin having results, stay at that dose for up to three weeks and then taper back gradually to 6 to 10 mg daily.

Manganese is another mineral deficient in diabetics. They tend to have about half the amount found in healthy individuals. Manganese helps key enzymes in the body utilize vitamin C and some B vitamins, as well as regulate glucose metabolism. Manganese supplements have reversed diabetes in guinea pigs. Not much research has been conducted in humans, but I personally know clinicians who have successfully treated insulin resistance by giving manganese along with chromium and zinc, in combination with diet and exercise. Consider taking 1 to 5 mg to prevent Syndrome X, but if you have high documented glucose levels or any other symptoms of Syndrome X, up to 10 mg may be needed. Take this separately from calcium.

Selenium, at 100 to 200 mcg daily, helps antioxidants do their job more effectively. It helps boost immunity and may play a role in preventing heart disease and cancer. Take with vitamin E.

ANTIOXIDANTS

Alpha lipoic acid, a nutritional supplement available over-the-counter, is a super antioxidant that fights the injuries inflicted by free radicals, those unstable molecules that are byproducts of cell activity. Excessive amounts of free radicals can damage cell structures, impair the immune system, cause inflammation and ultimately contribute to most chronic and degenerative diseases. What is unique about alpha lipoic acid is that it is both fat and water soluble, which enhances its ability to trap free radicals.

Alpha lipoic acid holds promise as a treatment and preventive for nerve damage complications faced by people with diabetes. More than 200,000 deaths a year can be attributed to nerve damage as the result of elevated blood glucose levels. Nerve damage is responsible for increasing diabetics' risk of leg amputations by up to 40 times more than the general population, it is also the leading cause of blindness among adults, and is associated with kidney diseases. Studies show that alpha lipoic acid can prevent or slow nerve damage experienced by up to 70 percent of diabetics, and there is even evidence that it can slow the aging process.

Research in Germany—where alpha lipoic acid has been used to treat diabetic nerve damage for more than 30 years—shows that diabetics taking 600 mgs of alpha lipoic acid daily experienced a reduction in nerve damage-related pain and numbness. Other work by German researchers has shown that alpha lipoic acid enhances the action of insulin and antidiabetes drugs in lowering blood-glucose levels.

Alpha lipoic acid can help prevent Syndrome X at levels as low as 50 mg per day, preferably as part of a multivitamin or antioxidant supplement that also contain vitamins E and C and other antioxidants. Take doses ranging from 100 to 300 mg to reverse problems related to glucose intolerance and insulin resistance. The recommended daily dose in Germany for diabetics suffering from nerve damage is 600 mg, but this amount should be taken under the guidance of a health care professional. Higher doses may reduce requirements for medications that lower glucose levels.

Vitamin E, like alpha lipoic acid, is an important antioxidant that counteracts many of the negative effects of free radicals, thereby reducing the disease-promoting effects of diabetes. In fact, two independent studies have shown that low blood levels of vitamin E are correlated with a four times higher risk of diabetes. Vitamin E protects cells from the harmful effects of glucose, reduces glucose levels, improves insulin sensitivity, and slows the aging process and age-related diseases. As an antioxidant, vitamin E prevents LDL cholesterol from building up in the blood vessel walls and from oxidizing, thus neutralizing two key factors of heart disease. It also reduces the risk of blood clots and improves circulation. To help protect against diabetes, insulin resistance syndrome, and heart disease, take 400 IU of vitamin E daily in the form of mixed tocopherols.

Vitamin C is a powerful antioxidant that quenches free radicals formed by glucose and immune cells, reducing the damage that can cause heart disease and cancer. Additionally, vitamin C blocks many of the harmful effects of elevated glucose and insulin levels.

Interestingly, vitamin C and glucose have nearly identical chemical structures. This is good for most animals, but for humans the similarity causes confusion at the cellular level and increases the risk for diseases caused by elevated glucose. Most animals can convert glucose into vitamin C, but the same doesn't hold true for humans. Glucose and vitamin C compete in the human blood system, for both want to ride insulin to the cells. When a person becomes insulin resistant as a result of many years of glucose excess, that person conceivably also becomes resistant to vitamin C, so it isn't surprising that many diabetics are also deficient in vitamin C. In other words, insulin resistance interferes with how cells use glucose *and* vitamin C. Low levels of vitamin C are associated with diabetic complications, including heart disease, kidney disease, and eye disorder.

The good news is that supplementing vitamin C helps lower glucose levels and normalize insulin's response to glucose. Vitamin C also boosts the body's immune system so that it can fight infection, normalizes cholesterol levels, relaxes blood vessels, lowers blood pressure, controls free-radical activity and damage, and reduces the risk of blood clots. In a study published in the *Journal of Clinical Investigation,* researchers at Harvard who gave diabetic patients intravenous vitamin C found that it significantly improved blood vessel dilation and function. Since impaired blood flow is one of the primary causes of diabetes complications, this is a significant finding.

To increase your protection against insulin resistance syndrome and for general well-being, take 1,000 to 2,000 mg of vitamin C daily. Double this amount to reverse insulin resistance. Some nutritionists recommend 3,000 to 6,000 mg a day. Make sure you're getting your citrus or rosehip bioflavonoids to help absorb the vitamin C. **Note:** Vitamin C can give false reading on some types of glucose tests, so consult with your physician or pharmacist about which form of glucose testing works best with vitamin C.

Bioflavonoids are not vitamins in the strictest sense but are sometimes referred to as vitamin P. As an antioxidant and doubling as color pigments for the plants, they protect against free radicals. They are useful in promoting circulation, lowering cholesterol, protecting against bruising, relieving leg pains and cramps, and preventing or treating eye disease. Bioflavonoids also have antinflammatory and anti-bacterial properties. A cup of green tea or a handful of berries can contain dozens of different bioflavonoids. Our ancestors probably consumed 1,000 mg of bioflavonoids a day, while Americans, who do not typically eat fruits and vegetables, consume maybe only 23 to 170 mg a day. Bioflavonoids enhance the absorption of vitamin C and the two should be taken together. Some useful bioflavonoids include:

- **Grape seed extract** works as an antioxidant and anti-inflammatory to help the body maintain levels of vitamins C and E. It strengthens connective tissue, including in the cardiovascular system.

- **Citrus bioflavonoids**, found in oranges, lemons, and grape fruit, have a beneficial effect on blood-vessel walls.
- **Green tea**, another powerful antioxidant, lowers cholesterol, strengthens blood vessel walls, fights infection, and may also lower blood pressure.
- **Quercetin**, a bioflavonoid found in onions and apples, can help people with diabetes because of its ability to reduce levels of sorbitol—a sugar that in diabetics accumulates in nerve cells, kidney cells, and in the eyes. It can also be effective in reducing allergy symptoms. You can take it as a supplement, 500 mg per day.

Carotenoids, like bioflavonoids, are the colorful plant pigments that pull double duty as antioxidants. More than 600 carotenoids have been identified, 50 of which are present in the Western diet, but only 14 of which are absorbable in the bloodstream. The most prominently researched is beta-carotene, which is converted to vitamin A in the body. One study showed that women taking 9,000 IU of beta-carotene were protected against LDL oxidation in the blood. It also activates different types of immune cells, which is important because glucose interferes with immune function, making diabetics more susceptible to infections. While beta-carotene won't correct glucose problems, it can bolster the immune system to offset glucose-related cellular damage.

The best way to get beta-carotene is by eating a vegetable-rich diet. If you wish to take it in supplemental form, know that natural beta-carotene, usually derived from D *salina* algae, is a more potent anti-oxidant than the synthetic version. Consider taking a supplement that combines natural beta- and alpha-carotene, lutein, and lycopene. Many diabetics are unable to convert beta-carotene to vitamin A in the body, and instead supplement with vitamin A.

Vitamin A, an essential nutrient and antioxidant, has been found to promote insulin sensitivity, because of its hormone-like effects. Vitamin A is also needed to maintain healthy eyes. Vitamin A is typically contained within a good multivitamin. If you do not take a multivitamin, consider taking 10,000 IU of vitamin A daily. Use an emulsion form for better absorption.

Coenzyme Q10, or **CoQ10,** is another antioxidant, but its key role is in efficient energy production at the cellular levels. The fuel for most of this energy is glucose, and CoQ10 helps the body metabolize carbohydrates, the source of glucose. It improves circulation and helps to normalize glucose levels. It also stops the early stages of heart disease by preventing oxidation of LDL cholesterol, reduces blood pressure and increases HDL cholesterol. It can also strengthen the heart, and prevent heart failure. Doses commonly range between 30 and 400 mg (the higher doses are more appropriate for heart patients).

OTHER IMPORTANT SUPPLEMENTS FOR STABLE BLOOD SUGAR

Vitamin D is required for the secretion of insulin by the pancreas. Studies now link a vitamin D deficiency with diabetes, immune function, bone loss and various types of cancer. It may be that vitamin D deficiency is a factor in the onset of diabetes and that a supplement of vitamin D could help reverse the disease. Spending just 15 minutes in the sunshine will help stimulate your body's own production of vitamin D. If you do not take a multivitamin, consider taking 400 to 2,000 IU daily.

B-complex vitamins are also essential for diabetics and anyone suffering from insulin resistance syndrome. B vitamins work best when taken together, so consider taking a B-complex vitamin. Your health care provider may want to pinpoint certain acute symptoms with specific B vitamins. These will be addressed separately:

Vitamin B6 is low in many diabetics, lower still in diabetics with nerve damage. Vitamin B6 supplements improve glucose tolerance in women with diabetes that occurs during pregnancy, and is also effective for treating glucose intolerance caused by birth control pills.

Vitamin B12 absorption is inhibited by most of the oral diabetes drugs. If you are taking these drugs, take B12 or a B-complex vitamin. In studies, vitamin B12 helped reduce nerve damage caused by diabetes. Take oral or sublingual vitamin B12, 1,000 to 2,000 mcg daily.

Biotin is a B vitamin needed to process glucose. When people with insulin-dependent diabetes were given 16 mg of biotin per day for one week, their fasting glucose levels dropped by half. Similar results have been reported using 9 mg per day for two months in people with non-insulin dependent diabetes. Biotin may also reduce pain from diabetic nerve damage.

Niacin, a form of vitamin B3, works with chromium to reduce nerve damage, and can be taken in the form of inositol hexanicotinate. To start, you can take 100 mg of niacin daily. For example, one brand of 500 mg tablets of inositol hexanicotinate yields 400 mg of inositol and 100 mg of niacin. You can gradually raise the dose if needed, up to 400 mg of niacin daily.

Methylsulfonylmethane (MSM), a form of organic sulfur, is another supplement that shows great potential in helping to stabilize blood sugar. You can take 1,000 mg two to three times daily. It works best when combined with vitamin C.

ESSENTIAL FATTY ACIDS (EFAS)

Omega-3 fish oil supplements improve glucose tolerance in *healthy* people, according to some studies, while other studies find that omega-3 fish oil improves glucose tolerance, high triglycerides, and cholesterol levels in diabetics. In one trial, people with diabetic neuropathy and diabetic nephropathy (kidney damage) experienced significant improvement when given 600 mg three times per day of purified EPA—one of the two major omega-3 fatty acids found in fish oil supplements—for forty-eight weeks. Most sources suggest 1 to 3 grams of fish oil capsules with meals per day. Be sure that it is well preserved and not rancid, and if you're experiencing fishy-tasting burps, stop taking them and eat more of the real thing!

Evening primrose oil has been found to reverse diabetic nerve damage and improve this painful condition, with 4 grams per day for six months. In double-blind research, 6 grams per day helped reduce nerve damage in people with both insulin-dependent and non-insulin-dependent diabetes.

Gamma-linolenic acid (GLA), an omerga-6 fatty acid, helps maintain normal nerve function and forms part of the sheath that coats the lengths of nerve cells. When omega-3 and omega-6 fats become unbalanced, or when overall fat levels are too low from low-fat diets, these sheaths become damaged, and nerve cells can't function properly.

The human body should make GLA from the linoleic acid found in grains, nuts, and other foods, but unfortunately, sugar, alcohol, hydrogenated trans-fats, and diabetes interfere with the activity of the enzyme that plays an important role in converting linoleic acid to GLA. Trans-fatty acids also interfere with the enzymes needed by the body to convert another omega-3 fat called docosahexaenoic acid (DHA). Most people benefit from 150 to 250 mg of GLA daily; diabetics, however, generally need up to 400 mg.

THE BENEFITS OF CARNITINE IN WEIGHT LOSS

The amino acid carnitine may be helpful in enhancing your body's ability to burn fat. Our bodies can make carnitine from the amino acid lysine, which is found in whole grains, legumes (including soy), and meats. To manufacture carnitine, your body also needs vitamin B6, niacin, iron, and vitamin C, so it's important to make sure you have enough of these nutrients. A deficiency of carnitine can cause fatigue, muscle weakness, heart disease, acidic blood, high triglyceride (fat) levels in the blood, and brain degeneration.

One of carnitine's primary jobs in your body is to carry fats across cell membranes into your cells' power plants, called mitochondria. There the fat supplies energy for many functions, especially the contraction of muscles. (Here is the ideal way to get rid of fat: transform it into fuel by burning it off with exercise!) When carnitine is plentiful in your body, more fat can be transported into your cells to be burned for energy. Some researchers also suggest that carnitine allows you to exercise longer without becoming fatigued.

Obviously, this fat-burning action makes carnitine a terrific supplement to help you lose weight, but it has other important benefits. For instance, it cleans up waste substances in the blood, which are formed when your body breaks down fat. Evidence shows that carnitine improves your liver's ability to break down fats for excretion. It can lower your blood levels of triglycerides (fats) and LDL cholesterol, and raise your levels of HDL cholesterol.

Carnitine comes in several forms, which you can find at your health food store. I recommend either L-carnitine, acetyl L-carnitine, or L-acetylcarnitine. The acetylated forms may be more easily absorbed, but they also tend to be more expensive. Read the labels on carnitine supplements carefully before you buy them. Please don't take the synthetic "D" or "DL" carnitine, because they can have negative side effects. Carnitine comes in tablets or capsules, usually 250 mg or 500 mg to burn fat, and for improved brain function, I recommend taking 1,000 to 2,000 mg daily on an empty stomach, in divided doses: (Take 500 mg two to four times a day.) To use carnitine for maintenance and prevention, take 250 to 500 mg daily.

Vitamin C greatly enhances your body's ability to use carnitine, so be sure you're getting at least 1,000 mg of vitamin C daily (which I recommend anyway) when you're taking it. Please be aware that carnitine's ability to improve alertness and attention may cause insomnia in some people. If this happens to you, try taking your last supplement half an hour before dinner.

Food-Specific Remedies for Glucose and Insulin Control

Onions, raw or cooked can lower blood sugar.

Garlic is a drugstore in and of itself. Not only can regular use control blood sugar, it reduces death from heart attack as much as 66 percent by the third year of taking it, and reduces high blood pressure and blood cholesterol by 10 percent. A steady infusion of garlic helps wash away arterial plaque and prevents future damage. Garlic can also reduce joint pains, body aches, and asthma, and improves vigor, energy, libido, and appetite. Raw garlic can irritate the stomach in some people, so if you're new to it, proceed with caution at first. You can eat one or two cloves of garlic daily, or take an aged, odorless garlic supplement of about 500 mg daily.

Barley bread, cabbage, lettuce, turnips, beans, juniper berries, alfalfa, and **coriander seeds** are among the 400 plant remedies that have been used to control blood sugar in Europe, Asia, and the Middle East for centuries. Modern tests confirm that all of them, or parts of them, can lower blood sugar or stimulate insulin production.

Jerusalem artichokes, burdock, and **parsley** are high in inulin, a fructose-like phytochemical that behaves like insulin.

Broccoli, Brewer's yeast, lean beef, calf's liver, whole wheat bread, wheat bran, rye bread, oysters, and **potatoes** are rich in chromium.

Oysters, ginger root, wheat germ, lamb chops, pecans, Brazil nuts, and **split peas** are rich in zinc. Paying attention to zinc intake is especially important for people who live in rainy coastal regions and prefer to eat locally grown foods. This is because the rainfall tends to wash trace minerals in the soil out to the sea, and minimal levels are absorbed into the produce.

Spices used in India to help control diabetes include **cinnamon, turmeric, bay leaf,** and **clove**. Turmeric and the more familiar spice cinnamon have both shown tremendous potential in helping regulate blood sugar. Test tube studies have shown that they triple insulin's ability to metabolize sugar.

Fenugreek is another herb that can help control your glucose levels.

Maitake mushrooms have been found to help maintain balanced blood sugar.

Aloe vera juice can help lower blood sugar levels.

CHAPTER 10

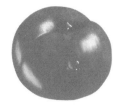

What's Keeping You from Optimal Health

UNLOCKING YOUR NATURAL ENERGY

IT'S MUCH MORE DIFFICULT TO GET UP off the couch and go for a brisk walk if your get-up-and-go has got-up-and-went. In other words, if you want to create a lifestyle that will create optimal health, energy, and weight loss, you need the energy to put that into motion. There are dozens of factors that can sap your energy, but in this chapter I'm going to cover the most common.

A friend of mine called a few months ago, complaining that she was feeling tired all the time, having trouble sleeping, and getting frequent colds. She is a working mother with two young children, and although her husband works part time and spends the rest of his time taking care of the kids and the house, she still feels a lot of pressure to perform at work, and never feels as if she's spending enough time with her kids. Her relationship with her husband wasn't a very happy one either, mainly because she felt she didn't have anything left to give to her relationship with him. In other words, stress was her way of life and her adrenal glands were probably close to exhausted. She's also in her early forties, an age when many women's hormone levels are beginning to drop, which can cause symptoms of fatigue, achiness, and irritability.

I told her my guess was that vitamin B12 shots and some progesterone cream would be a good beginning, but referred her to a doctor I know who incorporates nutrition, herbs, and other "alternative" forms of medicine into his practice. My friend called me few days later and said, "Sure enough, he put me on B12 shots and progesterone cream. He also gave me some herbs and supplements, and I'm scheduled to get a massage tomorrow. And he read me the riot act about not eating sugar." She called a few months later to thank me, saying she felt like a new woman, and she hadn't had so much energy since before she had her kids.

Does this all sound familiar to you? If you feel as though you don't have as much energy as you would like, you're not alone. Fatigue is one of the most common complaints heard by health professionals. Unfortunately, most doctors won't be able to help you. The solutions are too simple! Yes, that's right. I have some very simple ways for you to boost your energy levels. However, I'm going to ask you to give up or cut down on some things that you may have a lot of resistance to letting go of. Like sugar. And coffee. As far as I'm concerned, they are America's two favorite drugs and America's two biggest energy drains.

Why Does Sugar Drain Your Energy?

Here's a partial list of what sugar does to your body:

- Suppresses the immune system
- Generates free radicals
- Contributes to obesity
- Upsets glucose and insulin balance
- Contributes to diabetes
- Causes hypoglycemia with its symptoms of fatigue, irritability and weakness
- Contributes to candida, an overgrowth of yeast in the body
- Raises triglycerides, a type of blood fat associated with heart disease
- Damages the kidneys
- Contributes to gallstones by raising cholesterol content of bile
- Causes premature aging
- Upsets the acid balance in the stomach
- Contributes to arthritis
- Increases cholesterol
- Interferes with the utilization of protein
- Makes food allergies worse
- Sorbitol causes diarrhea and irritable bowel syndrome in some people

Sugar Depletes Or Interferes with the Absorption of:

Vitamin C

B-complex vitamins

Chromium

Copper

Calcium

Magnesium

Sugar Facts

- The average person in America eats 133 pounds of sweeteners a year.
- The average American teenager eats 300 pounds of sugar a year.
- You would have to eat 30 yards of sugar cane to get the sugar you consume in one can of cola.
- There are the equivalent of 9 teaspoons of sugar in a can of cola.
- Some 20 to 25 percent of America's daily calories are consumed in sugar (nutritionally empty calories).
- Brown sugar is not healthier — it is simply white sugar with molasses or burnt sugar added.

10 WAYS TO INCREASE YOUR ENERGY

1. Cut down or cut out the sugar. Sugar quickly and temporarily raises blood sugar. Our bodies have a built-in sugar regulator, but they aren't designed to handle the intense concentrations of sugar we get when we eat a pastry or drink a soda. You're probably familiar with that rush of energy, or sense of well-being after you eat sugar. But within half an hour to an hour after eating sugar, blood sugar plummets. This signals the brain to turn on the adrenal glands, which try to get the blood sugar back up, but in the process adrenaline is released too. Adrenaline is the substance that, when we lived in caves, gave us the "fight-or flight" response. It's our way of coping with a sudden fright or stress. Our hearts beats faster, our blood pressure rises, our muscles prepare for action and our blood leaves our digestive system for other more survival-oriented parts of our body. When this happens regularly, the adrenal glands become exhausted.

Our blood sugar often ends up below what it was before we ate the sugar. This plunge, along with the adrenaline surge, can cause fatigue, weakness, shakiness, dizziness, "spaciness," headaches and irritability. So, we reach for more sugar, to get our blood sugar back up, and pretty soon we're looking for our next sugar fix every hour or so. Meanwhile, the precipitous rise and fall of our blood sugar has a chain reaction all over the body, causing imbalances ranging from too much acid in the stomach to too much cholesterol in the bile and a depletion of essential vitamins and minerals.

If you have problems with fatigue, the first thing I would recommend is that you wean yourself from white sugar. I realize this may seem impossible, but you can start by substituting fruit when you feel the need for sugar. If your energy is much better after a couple of weeks without white sugar, try cutting back on the very sweet fruits, and see if your energy picks up even more. Substitute less sugary fruits such as grapefruit and apples, and complex carbohydrates such as nuts, seeds, and whole grains. These foods will boost your energy more slowly, and your blood sugar won't plummet back down an hour later.

Most alcohol contains sugar, and many people who drink too much are also addicted to sugar. Increasing your energy may be as simple as eliminating alcohol from your diet.

2. Cut out or cut down on the coffee. There I go again, coming out against another of American's most treasured drugs: coffee. A study published in the *Annals of Internal Medicine* tested the effects of caffeine on healthy people. They found that after ingesting the equivalent of 2 to 3 cups of coffee, people felt "hypoglycemic" but when tested, their blood sugar levels were normal. The researchers speculate that the caffeine increases your brain's need for sugar, while at the same time it restricts it by constricting blood vessels and reducing blood flow. This would be enough to trigger the symptoms of hypoglycemia, prompting you to reach for a doughnut or candy bar. Try drinking tea instead. By the way, cutting out the coffee can be challenging. You may feel groggy and have a headache for a few days, but hang in there, because once that passes, I promise you'll feel much, much better! Remember to drink plenty of water while you're cutting out sugar and coffee.

3. Test for food allergies and sensitivities. If getting off sugar and coffee doesn't help boost your energy level, try an elimination diet to test for food allergies. Food allergies are a common cause of fatigue. The most common offenders, which I call the big three, are wheat, corn, and dairy products.

4. Balance your hormones. When Laura began getting the hot flashes and night sweats typical of a woman entering menopause, she visited her doctor. He gave her a prescription for PremPro, a combination of hormones that he said would solve her problems. While her hot flashes and night sweats did stop, within a few months she was almost constantly tired and bloated, her breasts were painful, she was irritable and moody, she was having trouble sleeping at night, and had gained more than ten pounds. When she went back to her doctor with these complaints, he dismissed her concerns about the hormones and gave her three more prescriptions: a diuretic to help with the bloating, a sleeping pill, and a diet pill. After she started taking those she added terrible headaches, memory loss, heart palpitations, and dizziness to her list of problems, and she could hardly get out of bed. After a few weeks of complete misery, she threw away all the drugs. She figured that hot flashes and night sweats were better than all the side effects of the drugs! Laura didn't have to suffer through menopause, and I'll tell you more about natural hormone balance shortly. Suffice it to say that millions of women have endured what Laura did, but many didn't know enough to throw the drugs away. There are a myriad of underlying causes of fatigue, and hormonal imbalance is among the more common.

Middle-aged women complain of fatigue more than any group. This is often caused by a syndrome called "estrogen dominance," which can be caused by many conditions, but is highlighted by a deficiency of the hormone progesterone. For details on creating hormonal balance, read the books *What Your Doctor May Not Tell You About Premenopause,* and *What Your Doctor May Not Tell You About Menopause* by John R. Lee M.D. and Virginia Hopkins.

5. Balance your thyroid. Low thyroid, called hypothyroidism, may be one of America's hidden epidemics and a major cause of fatigue. The thyroid replacement drug Synthroid is the top-selling prescription drug in the U.S.

Unfortunately, hypothyroidism is probably underdiagnosed. Many people, especially women, have a normal thyroid blood test but have low thyroid symptoms that are resolved when they take a thyroid supplement.

A good way to find out if your thyroid is low is to take your basal body temperature, which means to take it first thing in the morning, before you even sit up in bed. If you take your temperature under your arm, normally it should range between 97.8 to 98.2 degrees Fahrenheit, first thing in the morning. If your basal body temperature is below 97, there's a very good chance your thyroid is low. A woman's temperature fluctuates according to her menstrual cycle. It rises just after she's ovulated, and drops again just before she menstruates. The best time for a woman to take her basal body temperature is in the first few days after menstruation begins. If you want to know more about your thyroid and hypothyroidism, I recommend the book, *Hypothyroidism: The Unsuspected Illness,* by Broda O. Barnes, M.D., and Lawrence Galton.

6. Lose some weight. It was inevitable that I'd get to weight, wasn't it? Being overweight is a big energy drain. If you don't believe me, take a backpack, put a 10-pound bag of something like dog food or potatoes in it and carry it around all day. Gets pretty tiring, doesn't it? Most of us are about 20 pounds overweight.

7. Manage your stress. Working long hours, difficult relationships with co-workers or family members, lack of sleep, and unresolved emotional issues are a few of the stressors that many people cope with every day. Regardless of how healthy you are, constant stress will eventually take its toll on your energy levels. One of the best ways to combat stress is to learn a meditation technique of some kind. My meditation technique is to take a stroll in a beautiful little park that's located in a retreat center. I have a friend who takes a yoga class three times a week, and another who gets a massage every week with a person who lights a candle and puts on soothing music during the session. If you lead a stressful life, it's important to take a break that is just for you at some point during the day even if it's just a bubble bath. Notice what kinds of activities make you feel restored and peaceful, and do more of them. It can be very healthy to turn off the TV at night and spend time with family, friends, or even by yourself! Turning off the TV can also be a simple technique for getting to sleep earlier.

The word stress has its roots in the Latin for "narrow" or "tight." Have you ever felt the pressure of anxiety? Does your schedule keep getting tighter and tighter? Mental constriction is a familiar form of stress that is often expressed in the body.

External pressures from career, relationships, and finances, for example, are often considered causes of stress. But the true origins of stress lie in our personal *reactions* to external factors. The mind has a tremendous capacity for retraining. People do lose the urge to smoke, drivers do stay calm in the face of road hogs and even the boss has a lighter side to appreciate. Learn to relax your mind as well as your body and you will release the habitual thought patterns and responses which actually create stress.

8. Try the "green" drinks. At your local health food store you'll usually find an array of high-chlorophyll drinks such as spirulina, blue-green algae, wheat grass, and barley grass. These drinks help bring more oxygen into your system, as well as lots of highly absorbable vitamins and minerals. They can be a nice afternoon pick-me-up. One of my favorites is a fresh juice with apple juice, papaya, lime, and spirulina.

9. Try some ginseng. One of my favorite afternoon drinks is a cup of ginseng tea. This herb, which has been used by the Chinese for thousands of years as a tonic and rejuvenator, has been dubbed an "adaptogen." This means that whatever is out of balance in the body, ginseng will tend to help it balance out. It can help regulate blood sugar, support the adrenal glands, and help us feel more physically and mentally alert. There are a number of different kinds of ginseng. The most common are *Panax* (Chinese, Korean, and American varieties) and *Eleutherococcus* (Siberian). The best way to take ginseng is as a tea.

10. EXERCISE! It's amazing what a simple walk can do for your energy. Exercise gets the blood circulating, the lymph system moving, and generally perks up your body's ability to do it's job at keeping you healthy and happy. You may feel too tired to take a walk, but if you get up and do it anyway, you'll probably start feeling better very shortly. If you usually work out indoors, try to get some outdoor exercise, too. Your mother was right about fresh air and sunshine being good for you! (I'll talk more about exercise in the next chapter.)

ALLERGIES ARE AN ENERGY DRAIN

Spring is a fresh, exuberant time of year, with balmy breezes, green grass sprouting, and flowers blooming everywhere. But if you are allergic to pollens and grasses, as one in ten Americans are, spring may only mean sniffling and sneezing to you. Then, of course, there are summer and fall allergies too, as well as indoor allergies to dust, mold, and pets, and allergies to perfumes and other scented products. Since pollen is one of the most common causes of allergies, let's take a closer look at it.

WHY DOES POLLEN MAKE US SNEEZE AND SNIFFLE?

The body's reaction of sinus congestion and sneezing is the first sign that our immune system is reacting, or sensitive, to something in the environment. It's helpful (if not pleasant!) when our bodies fight off a real invader such as a virus or bacteria with an immune reaction, which we call a cold or flu. But when we react to pollens, it's annoying and can interfere with our enjoyment of life.

Once our immune system decides that a particular type of pollen is a hostile invader, it becomes "sensitized" to it, and can react with allergy symptoms for years, sometimes a lifetime. When spring arrives and the pollen begins to fly, our sensitized bodies release histamines, designed to fight the enemy pollen. In the process of attacking the invaders, the histamines cause inflammation and even damage tissues, causing sinus irritation, itchy eyes, and often lung irritation as well. Some people can develop rashes, eczema, or hives.

The often accompanying headaches and mental fogginess are caused by sinus congestion. Sneezing is caused by irritated sinuses. Sore throats are caused by the mucous that runs down the back of the throat and asthma can be triggered by an overload of irritants and mucous. If the body tries to rid itself of the invaders via the skin, rashes, eczema, and hives may result.

Allergy drugs work to suppress symptoms rather than treat the cause of the allergy. The consequences of this type of treatment are generally unpleasant side effects and often there's a rebound effect where the symptoms are worse if the medication starts to wear off or treatment is stopped.

The simplest way to avoid allergy symptoms is to avoid the offending allergens. However, if you're allergic to pollens and grasses and love the outdoors and fresh air, this isn't a practical solution. The next simplest way to deal with allergies is to drink plenty of clean water. I recommend drinking at least 6–8 glasses a day during allergy season. Water not only helps flush toxins out of the body and supports proper cell function, but as our water levels go down, our histamine levels go up. Drinking a couple of glasses of clean water can quickly reduce allergy symptoms. Here are some other things you can do.

Support your immune system. The reason some people suffer from allergies and others don't certainly has to do with genetic predispositions, but it also seems to have to do with how well your immune system is working. If you already have a weakened immune system from chronic nutritional deficiencies, disease, lack of exercise or other factors, you're much more susceptible to allergies.

The best way to support your immune system over time is to make my 10 Core Principles (see Chapter One) a way of life. In a nutshell, that means taking the recommended supplements, getting daily exercise, drinking plenty of clean water, and adopting a diet that's high in fiber, fresh fruits and vegetables, and low in "bad" fats, sugar, and processed foods. You can also support your immune system by getting enough rest, reducing stress, and avoiding drugs and alcohol. If you need some extra help, here are some natural remedies.

HERBS AND FOODS TO HELP BANISH ALLERGIES

Echinacea: Take two droppersful of the tincture (preferably the fresh extract) in water, or two capsules, three times daily. Don't take echinacea for more than two weeks at a time, or it will start to lose its effectiveness. Through allergy season, take it two weeks on, and two weeks off. Some people are allergic to echinacea, so if it makes symptoms worse, stop taking it!

Astralagus: This Chinese herb has been used by healers in that country for centuries to restore normal function to the immune system. Take one to three 400 mg capsules daily.

Shiitake and Reishi: These mushrooms are another Oriental remedy for supporting the immune system. They're expensive, but you don't need to use much—one or two small mushrooms per serving should do the trick. During allergy season add these to your diet at least once a week, or take in capsule form.

Garlic: the more I study and research garlic, the better it looks. If you like the taste, make it a part of your daily diet, and if you don't you can take it in capsule form. In addition to lowering cholesterol, lowering blood pressure, killing intestinal parasites, reducing the risk of blood clots, inhibiting some cancer tumors and aiding digestion, garlic is a potent antioxidant, helping the body keep our cells healthy, intact, and functioning smoothly.

Yogurt: If you eat yogurt with live cultures daily as I recommend, you may greatly reduce the severity of your seasonal allergy symptoms. A one-year study at the University of California at Davis showed that those who ate just under a cup of yogurt daily had significantly reduced hay fever symptoms and also suffered from fewer colds.

Milk Thistle *(Silybum marianum)* is an herb that's been used in folk medicine for centuries and is now gaining respect thanks to scientific studies. It has been clearly shown in studies to greatly support the liver, even to the extent of regenerating liver cells. Since your liver is one of the main places your immune system dumps toxins, it pays to support it during allergy season.

VITAMINS AND MINERALS THAT CAN HELP WITH ALLERGIES

Vitamin C: If I could only recommend one thing to help with allergy symptoms it would be vitamin C. Many Americans are deficient in this essential vitamin, which works directly to lower histamine levels in the body and supports the immune system in many ways. During allergy season I recommend you take at least 1,000 mg three times daily, and if your symptoms continue or worsen, increase the dose to 1,000 mg every two or three hours.

Beta carotene, vitamin E and the **B vitamins:** if you suffer from seasonal hay fever, double your intake of these vitamins, which all support immune system function.

Calcium and Magnesium: Both have been shown to reduce hay fever symptoms.

Quercetin: This is a powerful antioxidant flavanoid that has been shown to fight cancer tumors and seems to be very effective in helping to fight allergy symptoms. I like it best combined with bromelain.

DEPRESSION: IT'S NOT ALL IN YOUR HEAD

With very few exceptions, we all have cycles in our lives when we're down, cycles when we're up, and cycles when we're somewhere in between. For example, it's quite normal to feel some level of depression before, during, or after a major life change such as the death of someone close, illness or injury, birth, marriage, divorce, a job change, or a move. When we're very "high" or excited about something, we'll normally have a corresponding dip in our emotions. These emotional ups and downs are all part of being human, and most of us learn to cope with them pretty well by the time we're middle-aged. Debilitating depression that makes a person nonfunctional for weeks or months at a time is another story.

Minor depression can be a form of "time-out" for adults. Sometimes it's nature's way of giving us a rest, or a signal that it's time to look within ourselves and be reflective. Maybe it's a message from the psyche telling us we need to re-evaluate our lives. This re-evaluation is most often an inner call to align ourselves with a sense of purpose, or mission in life—to go for what we *really* want, to reach for our dreams, even if they seem completely out of reach.

Unfortunately, thanks to a massive, multimillion-dollar public relations campaign on the part of the giant pharmaceutical companies who sell drugs such as Zoloft, millions of people believe that if they aren't feeling wonderful all the time, they need to fix it by taking a pill. You need to be aware that these pills are expensive, addictive, and have serious side effects!

In my experience, I've come to learn that there's usually no single solution for depression—a multi-faceted approach usually works best. For example, about a year ago, an older friend called complaining of depression. His wife had died the year before, and he had gone downhill and hadn't been able to climb back up. I asked him if he had any support from friends or family. He said no, his family didn't live nearby, and his wife had taken care of their social life—he hadn't continued it. I asked him how he was eating. He said his wife had done all the cooking, and he was mostly eating TV dinners or out of cans. Was he taking any medications? Yes, he was taking beta-blockers for high blood pressure, and sleeping pills. Was he taking any vitamins or supplements? No. Was he getting any exercise? Other than mowing the lawn, no.

Do you get my drift here? I'll bet you already know what I suggested to my friend: that he get out of the house and lend a helping hand somewhere as a volunteer; that he call up friends and invite them for a walk or a meal; that he take some cooking classes and eat fresh, unprocessed foods; that he ask his physician for a different method of lowering his blood pressure or try natural methods since beta-blockers can cause depression; that he wean himself off the sleeping pills; that he follow my 10 Core Principles; that he take supplements; and that he find a way to get some exercise every day. I know this sounds like common sense—and it is—but when you're depressed, it's not always easy to see the obvious.

The first step is to get up out of bed, or off the couch, and *do* something. Anything. Sweep the floor, go for a walk in the park, get a haircut, call a friend. Getting up and moving is one of the great cures for depression. Giving to others, forgiving others, and remembering what you're grateful for helps too. I realize this is easier said than done when you're *in* the thick of it, but go ahead and do it anyway!

And by the way, I called my friend back and he told me that he asked an old friend to teach him how to cook, and now they're dating! They are swimming at the Y together a couple of times a week, and meeting in a nearby park for walks. He also donated an old computer to a retirement home, and goes there every week to teach residents how to use it. Many of them are now active on a Senior Citizen's online bulletin board. He's on a lower dose of beta-blocker and expects not to need them in the near future. He admitted it had taken him awhile to get off the sleeping pills, but he finally succeeded. So are you still depressed, I asked? "Heck no!" he said. "I'm too busy to be depressed!"

If you're depressed to the point of being nonfunctional for weeks or months at a time, and haven't had any luck with conventional medicine, try to find a reputable alternative health care professional or an M.D. who uses nutrition, supplements, or herbs in his or her practice. Very often, the skillful use of nutrition, supplements, and amino acids can help people whose depression is biochemically related.

THREE THINGS TO TRY BEFORE TAKING
A SEDATIVE OR ANTIDEPRESSANT DRUG

Many people have written me with horror stories about taking sedatives and antidepressants, and asked for alternatives. Let's face it, folks. Prescription drugs don't work very well for anxiety and depression, and they don't fall into my "safe" category. Unlike the FDA, I don't consider a medicine that has side effects at normal doses and is addictive to be "safe and effective." And one of the most common side effects of sedatives and antidepressants is depression! Some of the other most common side effects include impotence, drowsiness, insomnia, agitation and restlessness, irritability, and liver damage.

A HAPPY NATURAL REMEDY FROM THE SOUTH PACIFIC

If you're working on exercising and letting go of alcohol, sugar, or coffee, but want some gentle, natural help along the way in overcoming anxiety or depression, an herb called kava (*Piper methysticum*) might do the job for you. This member of the pepper family grows as a bush in the South Pacific. Kava root, ground up and mixed with coconut milk, is used by the South Pacific islanders in celebrations and ceremonies. If you've visited the South Pacific, you've probably been treated to a kava drink. Kava is described in medical terms as being a sedative and muscle relaxant, and in lay terms as a calming drink that brings on a feeling of contentment, well-being and encourages socializing. No wonder I've come to know the South Pacific Islanders as very easy to get along with! Kava is also a pain reliever, and can often be used in place of NSAIDS (non-steroidal anti-inflammatory drugs such as aspirin, acetaminophen and ibuprofen).

In Europe, numerous double-blind and placebo studies have consistently shown kava to be as effective in treating anxiety and depression as so-called anti-anxiety drugs, but without the side effects. Quite the opposite in fact. The benzodiazepines (e.g. Serax, Valium, Ativan) tend to cause lethargy, drowsiness, and mental impairment. But in one double-blind placebo study done with 84 anxious people taking 400 mg daily of kavain (a purified kavalactone, an active ingredient of kava), concentration, memory, and reaction time improved. Other studies have shown no mental depression or interference with the ability to do tasks such as driving a car. In another study, people with anxiety symptoms given a 70 percent kavalactone extract (100 mg three times a day) were found after four weeks to have a significant reduction in feelings of nervousness, heart palpitations, chest pains, headaches, dizziness, and indigestion. In medicinal doses, kava has no known side effects. In very high doses, it can cause sleepiness, and high doses over a long period of time can cause skin irritation.

There have been reports of liver damage caused by using high doses of kava—the solution is simple—follow the instructions on the bottle and don't mix it with other drugs.

The best way to take kava is powdered, in a capsule, or as an extract.

THE B VITAMINS

The B vitamins play an essential role in our neurological health, and yet most adult Americans are deficient in these vitamins. Although each of the B vitamins play some role in brain function, vitamin B12 is best known for its ability to combat depression. For years, alternative health professionals have given vitamin B12 shots as part of an overall treatment program for people who are stressed out or depressed.

Prescription Drugs that Can Cause Depression

One of the most common causes of depression is prescription drugs. Here is a list of some of the most common prescription drugs that can cause depression:

Amphetamines (including antihistamines)

Antibiotics

Anticonvulsants

Antidepressants (I kid you not)

Barbiturates

High blood pressure drugs (beta-blockers, diuretics)

Hormones (synthetic progestins)

Narcotics

Painkillers

Sleeping pills

Systemic corticosteroids (prednisone, cortisone, etc.)

Tagamet and **Zantec**

Tranquilizers (Halcion, Librium, Restoril, Xanax, etc.)

THE POWER OF SLEEP

What better way to end this potpourri of amazing natural remedies than with a good night's sleep! You've no doubt heard that you should be getting about eight hours each night, but did you know that adequate, restorative sleep is the primary determinant of longevity—more than even exercise or proper nutrition? Sleep deprivation weakens your immune system, increases your fatigue, impairs your concentration, and may make you more irritable, anxious, or depressed. While you sleep, your cells regenerate and recharge, your metabolism takes a much-needed break, and your brain reorganizes itself.

Unfortunately, many Americans are moderately to severely sleep-deprived. In our attempt to juggle work, family, friends and other commitments, we often end up sacrificing healthy slumber in the name of survival—but pay the price in diminished energy, health, and overall quality of life. Also, insomnia is an increasingly common complaint, especially among students, business travelers, shift workers, and others who keep irregular hours.

Clearly, restorative sleep is one of the best health remedies available—and it doesn't cost a cent. Here are some tips for getting enough sleep, night after night:

- Maintain a regular sleep-wake schedule. That is, go to bed and wake up at the same time every day, as much as possible.
- Avoid caffeine, chocolate, alcohol, and tobacco, which disrupt natural sleep rhythms.
- Get plenty of exercise, but not within three hours of bedtime.
- Sleep in a quiet, dark bedroom, and limit your bed to sleeping and sex.
- Develop a bedtime ritual that includes calming activities such as a warm bath, quiet music, meditation or other stress-reduction techniques. Avoid stimulating conversations or work-related reading right before bed.
- If you can't get enough sleep at night, take short naps in the afternoon at a regular time. Avoid long naps because they may cause nighttime insomnia.

When you wake up feeling rested and remain alert throughout the day, you know that your body is getting the sleep it requires.

CHAPTER 11

There's No Getting Away From It

EXERCISE IS THE BEST MEDICINE

DARLENE WAS NEARING SIXTY AND HAD been overweight for most of her life. Although type 2 diabetes ran in her family, Darlene had been in denial about her own risk of developing the disease. Occasionally, she'd drop a few of the excess pound, usually for a special occasion such as the marriage of her daughter or her high school reunion. The weight always came back—usually more than she'd lost—as soon as she quit her desperate dieting regime of meal replacement shakes, saltines, and salads.

At her yearly physical, Darlene's doctor warned her that she was insulin resistant and would likely become a diabetic if she didn't make some drastic lifestyle changes. Darlene agreed to follow the doctor's dietary advice to the letter. Although she said she'd start an exercise program, Darlene felt her heart sink when the doctor told her she would need to do so. She'd never been able to stick to any kind of workout regimen, and knew herself well enough to know that she probably wouldn't do so now.

She'd joined the gym on three separate occasions, and had let her membership lapse each time. To be honest, the taut young bodies clad in Spandex made her feel ugly and cumbersome, and she couldn't bear to keep going back. She'd been intimidated by the machines, and didn't know the first thing about how to get going and stay motivated. When a hard-bodied male trainer had come to her aid, he had treated her in such a condescending and bored fashion that she'd walked away feeling even worse. Besides, she didn't want to sweat. She didn't want to huff and puff with exertion. She didn't want to have sore muscles. Her knees had become mildly arthritic and she worried about making them worse. And she certainly didn't have money to pay a trainer or to buy hundred-dollar exercise shoes.

Does Darlene remind you of anyone you know? Overweight people are told they must exercise to control their weight and maintain their health, but are given little-to-no guidance beyond the edict, "Just do it." When people like Darlene seek out information about *how* to "do it," they are bombarded with advertising for the latest miracle exercise gadgets and workout shoes, with headlines shouting about exercises that firm, tone, and tighten in only minutes a day, and with TV infomercials that promise to make workouts easy, effective, and fun. It's hardly surprising that so many people give up on exercise again and again.

Unfortunately, for those who would much rather relax with a cool drink than sweat through an aerobics class or strain through an uphill walk, exercise is essential to a healthy lifestyle—there's no getting around it. Then the challenge becomes finding a form of exercise that's meaningful and enjoyable, and I'm firmly convinced that there's something for everyone. It may take some creativity and self-discipline on your part, but it will be well worth the effort. Recent studies have shown that people who start an exercise program in response to a doctor's request don't stick with it. I suggest that you make an attitude adjustment that has you thinking of exercise not as a matter of choice in your life, but a matter of routine that you wouldn't think of doing without, such as brushing your teeth in the morning or putting gas in your car.

Exercise and diet together have been proven to enhance weight loss and prevent weight gain, and have been shown to delay the onset of type 2 diabetes in susceptible people. In one study of 11 obese African-American women, a single week's worth of 50 minutes of moderate, daily aerobic exercise dramatically improved glucose tolerance. In five of the subjects, their insulin resistance completely went away!

If you're like Darlene, you'd heard all this before, and the question may still remain: How do I get started and stick with it this time? In this chapter, you'll find out how to simply, safely, and effectively add exercise to your life—for good. I'm not going to throw a lot of confusing numbers at you or tell you to tie yourself into a yogic knot; the advice you'll get will be refreshingly simply and clear.

HOW EXERCISE HELPS

Oxygen is the "spark" that metabolizes carbohydrates and fats for energy. During exercise, your muscles use up oxygen much more quickly than they do at rest. That's why you breathe faster, and that's why your heart pumps more quickly—to deliver needed oxygen to hard-working muscles so that they can metabolize carbohydrates and fats for energy.

Your body has an amazing, practically fail-safe system for getting fuel and oxygen to all of the tissues that need them during exercise, including mechanisms that move glucose into cells without the help of insulin. In other words, an exercising body can bypass insulin resistance. During a workout, blood insulin and glucose levels drop, and levels of insulin's opposing hormone, glucagon, rise. The positive effects of exercise on blood sugar balance can last for hours following a workout. A regular exercise program has also been shown to lower blood pressure, and may improve fibrinolysis—the body's ability to break apart blood clots that can clog blood vessels.

Needless to say, the benefits of exercise go far beyond improvements in the shape of your body. While regular exercise, along with wholesome food I recommend in this book, will most likely help you drop excess weight, don't expect it to morph your figure back to the way it looked when you were 20. Many hopeful new exercisers abandon their programs when they find their bodies don't change as much as they'd like. Think of the outward, cosmetic changes as bonuses, and the internal, life-extending, health-enhancing changes as the real benefits of exercise, and you won't have to struggle with unreasonable expectations.

BEFORE YOU BEGIN

It doesn't matter what your health is right at this moment: You can still do some exercise. Any movement is better than no movement. Even if you've just come out of surgery, your doctor should be encouraging you to get up and walk around. However, if you want to move into more strenuous exercise than you're used to, be sure that you don't have the following conditions:

- If a condition called *proliferative diabetic retinopathy* is found in your eyes, you should avoid any exercise that involves jarring, bouncing, or straining movements—including running, lifting heavy weights, or doing high-impact aerobics. Such activities could cause retinal detachment or *vitreous hemorrhage* (a burst blood vessel within the eye), both serious threats to vision.

- If your doctor finds that you have peripheral neuropathy caused by poor foot circulation, you will need to make a special effort to protect your feet while exercising. Feet with reduced sensation are more easily injured, and those injuries won't heal as quickly as injuries to other parts of your body. A simple blister or scratch can become infected and eventually lead to serious problems. In more severe cases of neuropathy, only non-weight-bearing exercises, such as swimming or stationary bicycling, are recommended. Anyone with type 2 diabetes should examine their feet after every workout, and keep their toenails well-groomed to prevent ingrown nails and hangnails.

• If lab tests reveal that your kidneys aren't functioning well, you may need to do only very gentle exercise in a professional rehabilitation setting.

Type 2 diabetics also should measure their blood sugars before and after every workout. While this may seem like a bit of a chore, you'll find it to be wonderful positive reinforcement when you see your sugars dropping consistently. Those who need to use insulin or medications may need to adjust their regimens if sugars are rising too high or dropping too low before, during, or after workouts.

THINGS YOU'LL NEED

Assuming that you're able to do weight-bearing exercise, your best bet is to begin walking. You can walk just about anywhere, and you don't need any exotic equipment to get going. If you don't already have the following, buy:

1. A pair of athletic shoes—running or cross-training—that have silica gel or air-filled midsoles. These midsoles will support your arches and protect your feet and legs against hard walking surfaces such as concrete or blacktop. This will probably be your most significant expense, but the shoes will last if you only use them for walking workouts.

2. A few pairs of all-cotton sport socks. These will absorb moisture and prevent blisters.

3. A water bottle that's comfortable to carry with you while you walk. Proper hydration is an essential part of blood glucose control in insulin resistant people and type 2 diabetics.

4. A watch, so that you can keep track of your workout time.

Finally, see if you can enlist a workout partner—preferably someone around your age and fitness level. The last thing you need is a spry, overachieving exercise companion who's going to push you beyond where you're comfortable or someone who's less motivated than you are and continually steers your walks down the street with the doughnut shop. You'll be amazed at how quickly a workout passes when you're lost in a good conversation. If you can't find a willing workout buddy, try carrying an MP3 player so that you can listen to your favorite music or a book on tape.

For those who can't do weight-bearing exercise—those with peripheral neuropathy, for example, or those with disabling arthritis—water exercise, chair exercise (where workouts are done seated in a chair), or stationary bicycling are good choices. If you'd rather not go to a gym to ride a stationary bike, buying one for your home may be the way to go.

GETTING STARTED

You've put on your sweats, laced up your shoes, and filled your water bottle, and the time has come to begin your workout. Now what?

Just get yourself out the door and start walking. Don't set any goals yet. Just get out there and stroll along at whatever pace feels good to you. If you live in a hot climate and you're sensitive to the heat, walk in the morning or evening. If you're really out of shape, be sure to choose a route that's relatively flat. As you walk, take some deep breaths and relax. Remember that your body was made to move. If exercise doesn't feel good yet, it's because your body hasn't been moving enough. It will feel good in time, if you stick with it.

Your first day, you might only do a 10-minute walk. That's fine—recent research has shown that even 10 minutes of exercise is better than nothing. Congratulate yourself for whatever you've done. For the next week or so, simply put on your gear and go for a walk at least once a day. Make it part of your daily routine. Increase the time walked if you like, but don't feel like you have to. Chances are you'll end up walking more, and that it will start to feel good.

Make your workout walk different from your window-shopping or stroll-in-the-park walk. Stand tall, with your head balanced over your spine, chin slightly tucked, shoulders relaxed. With each step, feel the toes of the back foot pushing off, and reach forward with the other foot for a long stride. Let your arms swing freely.

Once you've gotten through that first week, you can begin to build on and refine your program. Eventually, you'll want to take three to four walks a week, 30 to 60 minutes apiece, or you can do more frequent, shorter walks. Try to build up to 90 to 240 minutes (1½ to 6 hours total) of walking or other aerobic exercise per week. Of course, if you can't do that much, don't worry about it—and don't quit. Something is always better than nothing when it comes to exercise.

REMEMBER TO STRETCH

One you've finished your walk, do a few gentle stretches to finish off your workout.

Calf stretch. Find a step and stand on it so that your heels point towards the edge. Scoot your right foot back until the heel dangles off the edge, then slowly bend the left knee, keeping the right leg straight. Your right heel will press down and you'll feel a powerful stretch in the right ankle and calf. *Gently* hold this stretch for at least 30 seconds, without bouncing, and then switch feet.

Hamstring stretch. Sit on the edge of a chair, both feet planted firmly on the floor. Straighten the right knee and flex the right foot, so that the right heel rests on the floor in front of you and the right toes point up towards your chin. Sit up as tall as you can, then clasp your hands and rest them on your left thigh as you tilt forward, bending from the hips. Try to keep your back straight as you fold your torso towards your legs. You should feel a stretch in the back of the right thigh. Hold for at least 30 seconds before switching legs.

Quadriceps stretch. Still sitting on your chair, place both feet on the floor in front of you. Scoot your hips to the right side of the seat. Slide your right foot back past the right side of the chair's legs, until the laces of your right shoe are against the floor and your knee is pointing towards the ground. You should feel a stretch in the front of the right thigh and the right hip. Hold 30 seconds and switch sides.

HOW HARD SHOULD YOU WORK OUT?

The most difficult thing for most novice exercisers to figure out is how hard they should work—the *intensity* required to get the benefits they want. You don't have to work very intensely to prolong your life and control your blood sugar; but if you're serious about losing weight or improving your cardiovascular fitness, you'll need to work a little harder. While the most important thing is for you to get out the door, even if it's just to slowly stroll along, you may be ready to push yourself a bit harder once you've established your routine and discovered how enjoyable it can be.

Exercise scientists have come up with many different ways to measure intensity; the most commonly used is heart rate. The speed of your heart rate is generally a good indicator of how hard you're working, but it isn't easy to measure your pulse while you're walking. Many older people take medications that affect heart rate, preventing it from changing normally during exercise.

What I suggest is that you use the rating of perceived exertion (RPE) scale. The RPE is commonly used in physical therapy and cardiac rehabilitation; it allows you to evaluate the sum of sensations in your body as you exercise, and to assign your level of exertion a value of a scale of 1 to 10. If you were strolling very slowly along the beach sipping a cocktail, you'd be at 1; if you were sprinting up the side of a mountain, you'd be at 10. For maximum benefit, your RPE should be at between 13 and 16 for at least 15 minutes of your work-out. You'll be breathing hard, but you shouldn't be out of breath (you should be able to complete a sentence without feeling as though you're not getting enough air); you'll probably break a light sweat; and you'll probably feel like you're pushing yourself just a little beyond your comfort level.

The beauty of the RPE is that you don't have to adjust it as you become fitter. As you get into better shape, you'll be able to exercise at a higher intensity without increasing your rating of perceived exertion. If you stay within that 13 to 16 range, you'll always be challenging your body and improving its fitness level.

STRENGTH TRAINING

Today, we know that building and maintaining muscular strength is an important component of fitness. A regular walking program will tone your lower body, but it's a good idea to balance with some simple exercises to keep arm, shoulder, back, and abdominal muscles strong. You can do these exercises at home, two to four times a week. You can even do them while you watch TV. Perform each exercise slowly, so that your muscles are always supporting and controlling the weight you're lifting. Breathe steadily and deeply as you work. If you can't do the 10 to 20 repetitions recommended at first, that's fine. Start out with 2 reps if you have to, and patiently work your way up over a period of weeks. The key is to start wherever you are, and do whatever you can.

Canned food curls. Stand or sit with your arms hanging down your sides. Keeping your elbows next to your waist, curl the cans slowly up towards your shoulders and just as slowly back down. If you have light weights, of course, use those instead. Repeat 10 to 20 times total.

Overhead presses. Hold the cans or weights at shoulder level, elbows bent. Press your arms straight overhead without locking your elbows. Repeat 10 to 20 times.

Upper back strengthener. Sit at the edge of a chair, feet flat on the floor. Hold a can or weight in each hand. Tilt your torso forward from the hips so that there's about a 45 degree angle between your thighs and the front of your trunk, without rounding your back. Look out at the floor a couple of feet in front of your toes. Let the cans hang straight towards the floor. Lift your arms out to the sides as though they were wings, elbows first, palms down, as high as you can comfortably go. Release back down towards the floor. Be sure to only move the arms, keeping the rest of your body still. Repeat 10 to 12 times.

Abdominal strengthener. Lie on your back on the floor with your feet resting on the seat of a chair. Cross your arms over your chest or behind your head. Inhale deeply, and as you exhale press your lower back into the floor with your abdominal muscles. It will feel as though your belly button is pressing in towards your spine. Your hips will tilt up towards the ceiling as you do this. Release as you inhale. As you get stronger, you can begin lifting your shoulders and head slightly off of the floor as you press your lower back down. Keep your chin tucked into your chest as you lift your head. It's a very small movement, performed slowly and smoothly. Work towards 20 to 50 repetitions.

ADD ACTIVITY WHEREVER YOU CAN

Don't have time for a workout because you have company coming and you need to get the house straightened up? Go ahead and dust, mop, vacuum, and garden—and call it a workout. Need to go to the grocery store? Park your car at the far end of the lot and walk briskly through the aisles with your cart.

Feel like watching TV instead of going out for a walk? Pedal your stationary bike for the first half-hour of your program.

After all, in the days before obesity and blood sugar imbalances were epidemic, people weren't spending a whole lot of time in the gym. They were doing physical work—planting, harvesting, gathering, washing, walking, carrying, building—for much of every day. With all our modern conveniences, we're freed up from much of this physical labor, and our health has suffered. Adding a little activity here and there in your everyday life will make a huge difference in your health and fitness level.

Adrenaline: Also called *epinephrine;* a hormone released by the adrenal glands in response to stress, exercise, or strong emotion; chronic high levels can cause insulin levels to rise, causing eicosanoid imbalance.

Allergens: Substances that are normally harmless, but in certain conditions, produce an allergic reaction in some people.

Amino Acids: The building blocks of protein; they are classified into essential and non-essential amino acids.

Antigen: Foreign proteins which are recognized and attacked by the immune system.

Antioxidants: A substance that slows down oxidation and helps defend against free radicals. Oxidation is a chemical reaction with oxygen and can cause many diseases. They include vitamins C and E, carotenes and bioflavonoids.

Arachidonic Acid: A type of fatty acid, from which "bad" leukotrienes, thromboxanes, and prostaglandins are made with the help of enzymes (cyclooxygenases, thromboxane synthetase, and lipoxygenases).

Autoimmune disease: When the immune system attacks the body's own tissue, causing inflammation; rheumatoid arthritis, ulcerative colitis, lupus, and others fall into this category; thought to be attributable to standard Western processed-food diet.

Cartilage: Spongy, smooth tissue that provides cushioning between ends of bones; degeneration leads to osteoarthritis.

Cerebrovascular Insufficiency: A shortage of blood flow to the brain.

Chelation Therapy: An intravenous therapy that flushes heavy metals from the body with a solution containing a synthetic amino acid (EDTA).

Chondrocytes: Cartilage-making cells.

Collagen: The most abundant protein in the body; forms the framework for building of bone, cartilage, and other connective tissues.

Cortisol: Hormones secreted by the adrenal glands in response to stress, starvation, and exercise; chronic stress triggers high levels of cortisol, which can adversely affect eicosanoid balance.

Cyclooxygenases: Enzymes that transform activated fatty acids (GLA and DHGLA) into good or bad prostaglandins.

Cytokines: Immune cells that stimulate the inflammatory response. Interleukins (chemical messengers) that modulate the immune response and relieve inflammation; include IL-1, IL-6, and IL-10.

Delta 5-Desturase: Transforms activated fatty acids into eicosapentaenoic acid and arachidonic acid; a healthy diet decreases its activity, which improves eicosanoid balance by decreasing the formation of bad eicosanoids from omega-6 fats.

Delta 6-Desaturase: Transforms essential fats from the diet into activated fatty acids, GLA, and DHGLA; stifled by high cortisol and adrenaline levels caused by stress, which can disrupt eicosanoid balance.

Dementia: Refers to any general decline in mental ability.

Dihoma-Gamma-Linoleic Acid (DHGLA): An Activated fatty acid created when delta 6-desaturase acts on linoleic acids from omega-6 oils.

DNA/RNA: Chains of acids which are stored in cells and contain genetic information.

Duodenum: The very first part of the small intestine after the stomach; often affected by NSAIDs, developing ulcers or tears.

Eicosanoids: Short-lived hormones which act on the cells that make them or the cells in the immediate vicinity; consist of three groups: the prostaglandins, the leukotrienes, and the thromboxanes; have widespread effects on blood clotting, inflammation, blood pressure, pain, and the health of the immune and gastrointestinal systems; many drugs work by suppressing these hormones.

Eicosapentaenoic Acid (EPA): The healthful fat that is created when delta 5-desaturase and delta 6-desaturase enzymes act on omega-3 oils; is then transformed by cyclooxygenases and lipoxygenases to good prostaglandins and leukotrienes.

Endorphins: Chemicals made in the body that are natural painkillers and mood enhancers; ginger constituents suppress thromboxane synthetase, which has effect of enhancing endorphin production; this may partially explain ginger's effectiveness as a painkiller.

Essential Amino Acids: The nine amino acids you must get from your food supplements, because they are not manufactured by your body.

Essential Fatty Acids: Omega-6 and omega-3 acids, which must be taken in from diet for survival.

Free Radicals: Created during the process of breaking down food molecules for fuel, much as a car creates exhaust; also created during inflammatory process; destructive to cells unless quenched by antioxidants.

Gamma-Linoleic Acid (GLA): Linoleic acids from omega-6 fats that have been acted upon by delta 6-desaturase enzyme.

Gastric: Having to do with the stomach.

Helicobacter Pylori (h. phlori): Bacteria thought to cause many cases of gastric ulcer.

Hippocampus: This is a seahorse-shaped part of the brain that lies within the temporal lobe and seems to be where much of short-term memory takes place.

Hyaluronic Acid: A natural joint-protective compound, destroyed by free radicals created during inflammation.

Hydrochloric Acid (HCl): Strong Acid secreted by stomach to digest food.

Immunoglobulins (antibodies): Molecules that identify and lock on to antigens, labeling them for destruction by other immune components.

Inflammation: Immune response to infection or injury, where immune cells and fluid are brought to the area, causing swelling, heat and redness; if uncontrolled through proper eicosanoid balance, can damage tissues.

Insulin-like Growth Factors (IGFs): Produced by the liver in response to stimulation by growth hormone; raises energy, mood and helps with fat loss, muscle and bone gain, and blood sugar balance; body makes less with age.

Interferon: Biochemical that stops viruses from multiplying in the body.

Interleukins: Components of the immune system that play a role in causing or decreasing inflammation.

Lactoferrin: An iron-binding biochemical with antioxidant, anti-inflammatory, and anti-bacterial effects.

Leaky Gut: When food allergies lead to inflammation in the small intestines, small leaks can form; undigested food particles escape into the circulation, causing immune responses; these responses to the joints could be the cause of rheumatoid arthritis.

Leukotriene: A type of eicosanoid that affects immunity, mucus secretion, and muscle contraction.

Lipoxygenases: A group of enzymes responsible for the formation of good and bad leukotrienes.

Lymphocytes: Immune cells; play an important role in the inflammatory process.

Metabolic Processes or Metabolism: Various chemical and physical processes, which enable food to be utilized by the body and which provide energy for vital functions.

Minerals: A group of inorganic elements essential for human health. They are also basic components of the earth's crusts.

Motility: How quickly food moves through the digestive process.

Natural Killer Cell: A type of immune cell, especially good at killing off cancer cells.

Neurotransmitters: Biochemicals that are responsible for the transmission of nerve impulses.

Nitric Oxide: A chemical made in the body; relaxes muscles in blood vessel walls, allowing them to open.

Non-Essential Amino Acids: Amino acids which are manufactured by the body. Non-essential is a misnomer, since in fact they are necessary for the body's functioning.

NSAIDs: Nonsteroidal anti-inflammatory drugs; relieve pain and inflammation by affecting eicosanoid balance; ginger extract works through same mechanism.

Oleoresin: The sticky part of the ginger rhizome, within which lies most of its active ingredients.

Omega-3 Fats: Essential fats found in fish, walnuts, and flaxseeds; raw material for good eicosanoids.

Omega-6 Fats: Essential fats found in polyunsaturated vegetable oils, borage, evening primrose; raw material for good eicosanoids or bad, depending on action of enzymes.

Oxidation: The process whereby free radicals are created.

Parasite: An animal, plant, or microbe that lives in or on another organism and feeds off it, without contributing anything in return.

Pepsin: An enzyme secreted in the stomach to break down proteins; typical ulcer drugs decrease its action, adversely affecting digestion.

Peristalsis: The rhythmic contractions of the muscular walls of the GI tract, which moves food along and mixes it with digestive juices.

Phytochemicals: Health-supporting natural chemicals from plants (phyto=plant).

Platelets: Components of blood responsible for creating clots; pro-inflammatory eicosanoids also tend to make platelets more "sticky," increasing the thickness of blood and the likelihood that a clot will form.

Probiotics: "Friendly bacteria" that live in the gastrointestinal tract; manufacture B vitamins, complete breakdown of food, neutralize toxins and carcinogens, maintain proper environment for good digestion.

Prostacyclin: A "good" prostaglandin that thins the blood and dilates (opens up) blood vessels; users of Celebrex suppress its formation.

Prostaglandin: A type of eicosanoid that modifies pain responses, inflammation, body temperature, the constriction and expansion of vessels, blood clotting, and the health of the stomach lining.

Protein: A chain of amino acids. Most of your body consists of protein. It is an organic substance consisting of oxygen, nitrogen, carbon, and hydrogen.

Rhizome: A root that will bud into new plants if split and planted.

Serotonin: A neurotransmitter important for mood; may play a role in causing migraine headache because of its interactions with platelets and substance P, a chemical in the body that stimulates the sensation of pain.

Standardized: Used to describe herbal extracts that are made to consistently contain the same amount of active ingredients.

Substance P: A chemical in the body that stimulates the sensation of pain.

Sulfites: Preservatives and additives used in food to prevent decay and discoloration.

Synergistic: Having the ability to work better together than separately.

Synthetic: Artificial. Substances that do not occur naturally or that are synthesized in a laboratory.

T-Cells: White blood cells, an important part of the immune system.

Thromboxanes: Eicosanoids responsible for blood clotting and pain responses.

Thromboxane Synthetase: An enzyme needed to make thromboxanes; increased levels suppress endorphins, while decreased levels encourage endorphin formation.

Transit time: The amount of time it takes for the contents of a meal to pass through the gastrointestinal tract and out of the body; short transit times mean better colon health.

Vitamins: A group of organic nutrients, found in plants and animals, which the body needs for normal metabolism and well-being. With Few exceptions, they cannot be manufactured by the body.

REFERENCES

Chapter Two

Brewerton, T., M. Heffernan, and N. Rosenthal. 1986. Psychiatric aspects of the relationship between eating and mood. *Nutritional Review* 44 (Suppl. May 1986):78–88.

Eaton, S.B., S.B. Eaton III, and M.J. Konner. 1997. Paleolithic nutrition revisited: A twelve-year retrospective on its nature and implications. *European Journal of Clinical Nutrition* 51:207–216.

Ferro-Luzzi, A., and F. Branca. 1995. Mediterranean diet, Italian-style: prototype of a healthy diet. *American Journal of Clinical Nutrition* 61:1338S–1345S.

Giovannucci, Edward, et al. 1993. A prospective study of dietary fat and the risk of prostate cancer. *Journal of the National Cancer Institute* 85(19):1571–1579.

Helsing, E. 1995. Traditional diets and disease patterns of the Mediterranean, circa 1960. *American Journal of Clinical Nutrition* 61:1329S–1337S.

Milne, David B., and Phyllis E. Johnson. 1993. Effect of changes in short-term dietary zinc intake on ethanol metabolism and zinc status indices in young men. *Nutrition Research* 13:511–521.

Mindell, E., and V. Hopkins. 1998. *Prescription Alternatives*. New Canaan, Connecticut: Keats Publishing. 400–420.

Willett, W.C. 1995. Mediterranean diet pyramid: a cultural model for healthy eating. *American Journal of Clinical Nutrition* 61:1402S–1406S.

Chapters Four and Five

Burkitt, D., and H. Trowell. 1981. *Western Diseases: Their Emergence and Prevention*. Cambridge, Massachusetts: Harvard University Press.

Cabellero, B. 1987. Brain serotonin and carbohydrate craving in obesity. *International Journal of Obesity* 11:179–183.

Challem, Jack, Burton Berkson, and Melissa Diane Smith. 2000. *Syndrome X, the Complete Nutritional Program to Prevent and Reverse Insulin Resistance*, New York: John Wiley & Sons.

Chen Y.D. 1995. Why do low fat, high carbohydrate diets accentuate postprandial lipemia in patients with NIDDM? *Diabetes Care* 18(1):010–016.

Coulston, A., M. Greenfield, F. Kraemer, L. Tobey and G.M. Reaven. 1980. Effect of source of dietary carbohydrate on plasma glucose and insulin responses to test meals in normal subjects. *American Journal of Clinical Nutrition* 33:1279–1282.

Coulston, A.M., G.C. Liu, and G.M. Reaven. 1983. Plasma, glucose, insulin and lipid responses to high-carbohydrate, low-fat diets in normal humans. *Metabolism* 32:52–56.

Eades, Michael, and Mary Dan Eades. 1996. *Protein Power*, New York: Bantam.; paperback edition by Creative Paradox, LLC.

Eaton, S.B., S.B. Eaton III, and M.J. Konner, et al. 1996. An evolutionary perspective enhances understanding of human nutritional requirements. *Journal of Nutrition* 126:1732–1740.

Food and Agriculture Organization/World Health Organization. 1985. Energy and protein requirements. *WHO Technical Report* 724.

Food and Agriculture Organization/World Health Organization. 1997. Carbohydrates in human nutrition. *Joint Expert Consultation*, Rome, 8, 19, 27, 80–81.

Golay, A., A.L.M. Swislocki, Y.D.I. Chen, J.B. Jaspan, and G.M. Reaven. 1986. Effect of obesity on ambient plasma glucose-free fatty acid, insulin, growth hormone, and glucagon concentrations. *Journal of Clinical Endocrinological Metabolism* 63:481–484.

Holt, S.H., J.C. Miller, P. Petocz, and E. Farmakalidis. 1995. A satiety index of common foods. *European Journal of Clinical Nutrition* 49:675–690.

Holt, S.H., J.C. Brand Miller, and P. Petocz. 1996. Interrelationships among postprandial satiety, glucose and insulin responses and changes in subsequent food intake. *European Journal of Clinical Nutrition* 50:788–797.

Jenkins, David J.A., et al. 1981. Glycemic Index of foods: a physiological basis for carbohydrate exchange. *American Journal of Clinical Nutrition* 34:362–366.

Laws, A., and C.M. Reaven. 1992. Evidence for an independent relationship between insulin resistance and fasting plasma HDL-cholesterol, triglyceride and insulin concentrations. *Journal of International Medicine* 231:25–30.

Liu, C. C., A.M. Coulston, and G.M. Reaven. 1983. Effect of high-carbohydrate-low-fat diets on plasma glucose, insulin and lipid responses in hypertriglyceridemic humans. *Metabolism* 32:750–753.

Liu, G., A. Coulston, C. Hollenbeck, and G.M. Reaven. 1984. The effect of sucrose content in high and low carbohydrate diets on plasma glucose, insulin, and lipid responses in hypertriglyceridemic humans. *Journal of Clinical Endocrinological Metabolism* 59:636–642.

Maheux, P., J. Jeppesen, WI-I. Sheu, et al. 1994. Additive effects of obesity, hypertension and type 2 diabetes on insulin resistance. *Hypertension* 24:695–698.

Markovic, Tania P., Arthur B. Jenkins, Lesley V. Campbell, Stuart M. Furler, Edward W. Kraegen, Donald and J. Chisholm. The determinants of glycemic responses to diet restriction and weight loss in obesity and NIDDM. *Diabetes Care* 21(5):687.

Reaven, Gerald, Terry Kristen Strom, and Barry Fox. 2000. *Syndrome X, Overcoming the Silent Killer that Can Give You a Heart Attack*, New York: Simon & Shuster.

Reaven, G., A. Calciano, R. Cody, C. Lucas. and R. Miller. 1963. Carbohydrate intolerance and hyperlipemia in patients with myocardial infarction without known diabetes mellitus. *Journal of Clinical Endocrinological Metabolism* 23:1013–1023.

Reaven, G.M. 1988. Role of insulin resistance in human disease. *Diabetes* 37:1595–1607.

Reaven, G.M. 1995. Pathophysiology of insulin resistance in human disease. *Physiological Reviews* 75:473–485.

Salmerón, J. 1997. Dietary fiber, glycemic load, and risk of NIDDM in men. *Diabetes Care* 20(4):545.

Sears, Barry, and Bill Lawren. 1995. *The Zone*, New York: ReganBooks.

Steward, H. Leighton, Morrision C. Bethea, Sam S. Andrews, and Luis Balart. 1995. *Sugar Busters: Cut Sugar to Trim Fat*. New York: Ballantine Books.

Torjeson, P.A., K.I. Birkeland, S.A. Anderssen, et al.1997. Lifestyle changes may reverse development of the insulin resistance syndrome. *Diabetes Care* 20:26–31.

Trevisan, M., J. Liu, F.B. Hahsas, et al. 1998. Syndrome X and mortality: A population-based study. *American Journal of Epidemiology* 148:958–966.

Zavaroni, I., E. Dall'Aglio, E. Bonora, O. Alpi, M. Passeri, and G.M. Reaven. 1987. Evidence that multiple risk factors for coronary artery disease exist in persons with abnormal glucose tolerance. *American Journal of Medicine* 83:609–612.

Wolever, T.M.S. 1990. Relationship between dietary fiber content and composition in foods and the glycemic index. *American Journal of Clinical Nutrition* 51:72–75.

Wolever, T.M.S., D.J.A. Jenkins, A.A. Jenkins, and R.G. Josse. 1991. The glycemic index: methodology and clinical implications. *American Journal of Clinical Nutrition* 54:846–854.

Chapter Six

Young, V.R. 1992. Protein and amino acid requirements in humans. *Scandinavian Journal of Nutrition* 36:47-56.

Chapter Seven

Ascherio, A., and W.C. Willett. 1997. Health effects of trans fatty acids. *American Journal of Clinical Nutrition* 66(suppl):1006S–1010S.

Axelrod, L., K. Kleinman, et al. 1994. Effects of a small quantity of omega-S fatty acids on cardiovascular risk factors in NIDDM. *Diabetes Care* 17:37–44.

Boden, G., X. Chen and J. Ruiz. 1994. Mechanisms of fatty acid-induced inhibition of glucose uptake. *Journal of Clinical Investigation* 93:2438–2446.

Fanaian, M., J. Szilasi, L. Storlien, et al. 1996. The effect of modified fat diet on insulin resistance and metabolic parameters in type II diabetes. *Diabetologia* 39:A7.

Garg, A. 1998. High-monounsaturated-fat diets for patients with diabetes mellitus: A meta-analysis. *American Journal of Clinical Nutrition* 67(suppl):577S–582S.

Gumbiner, Barry, Cecilia C. Low, and Peter D. Reaven. Effects of a monounsaturated fatty acid enriched hypocaloric diet on cardiovascular risk factors in obese patients with type 2 diabetes. *Diabetes Care* 21(1):9.

Swiskiocki, A.M., Y.D. Chen, M.A. Golay, M. D. Cheng, and G.M. Reaven. 1987. Insulin suppression of plasma-free fatty acid concentration in normal individuals or patients with type II (non-insulin-dependent) diabetes. *Diabetologia* 30:622–626.

Chapter Eight

Bloomgarden, Z.T. 2000. Studies in type 2 diabetes: highlights from the 36th annual meeting of the european association for the study of diabetes. Jerusalem, Israel.

Haffner, S.M., et al. 2000. The global scope of diabetes and obesity-an epidemic in progress: paradise lost. *Circulation*, 101:975–980.

Kakuda, T., et al. Hypoglycemic effect of extracts from Lagerstroemia speciosa L. leaves in genetically diabetic KK-AY mice. Central Research Institute, Itoen, Ltd., Sagara-cho, Haibara-gun, Shizuoka, Japan.

Sadahiko, Ishibashi, et al. Screening of plants constituents for effect on glucose transport activity in ehrlich masticates tumour cells. Institute of Pharmaceutical Sciences, Hiroshima University School of Medicine, 1-2-3 Kasumi, Minami-Ku, Hiroshima, Japan.

Suzuki, Y, T. Unno, et al. 1999. Antiobesity activity of extracts from Lagerstroemia speciosa L. leaves on female KK-Ay mice. *Journal of Nutritional Science and Vitaminology* (Tokyo) 45(6):791–5.

Chapter Nine

Anderson, R.A., N. Chen, N.A. Bryden, et al. 1997. Elevated intakes of supplemental chromium improve glucose and insulin variables in individuals with type 2 diabetes. *Diabetes* 46: 1786–1791.

Assan, R., et al. 1996. Dehydroepiandrosterone (DHEA) for diabetic patients? *European Journal of Endocrinology* 135: 37–38.

Baskaran, K. 1990. Antidiabetic effect of a leaf extract from Gymnema sylvestre in non-insulin-dependent diabetes mellitus patients. *Journal of Ethnopharmacology* 30: 295–305.

Basualdo, Carlota G., et al. 1997. Vitamin A (retinol) status of first nation adults with non-insulin dependent diabetes mellitus. *Journal of the American College of Nutrition* 16(1):38–45.

Bode, Ann M. 1997. Metabolism of Vitamin C in Health and Disease. *Advances in Pharmacology* 40:334–44.

Ceriello, Antonio, et al. 1991. Vitami– E Reduction of protein glycosylation in diabetes: new prospect for prevention of diabetic complications? *Diabetes Care* 14(1):68–72.

Challem, Jack. 1996. Antioxidants might ease diabetic complications. *Medical Tribune* 18.

Chen, M.D., P.Y. Lin, W.H. Li., et al. 1988. Zinc in hair and serum of obese individuals. *American Journal of Clinical Nutrition* 48:1307–1309.

Dela, Flemming. 1996. On the influence of physical training on glucose homeostasis *Acta Physiologica Scandinavica*: 5–33.

Eriksson, J, and A. Kohvakka. 1995. Magneium and ascorbic acid supplementation in diabetes mellitus. *Annals of Nutrition and Metabolism* 39:217–223.

Jam, Sushil K., et al. 1996. Effect of modest vitamin E supplementation on blood glycated hemoglobin and triglyceride levels and red cell indices in type I diabetic patients. *Journal of the American College of Nutrition* 15(5):458–461.

———. 1989. Hyperglycemia can cause membrane lipid peroxidation and osmotic fragility in human red blood cells. *Journal of Biological Chemistry* 264(35):21340–21345.

Jacob, S., E.J. Henriksen, A.L. Schiemann, et al. 1995. Enhancement of glucose disposal in patients with type 2 diabetes by alpha-lipoic acid. *Arzneimittel-Forschung Drug Research* 45:872–874.

Jacob, S., R.S. Streeper, D.L. Fogt, et al. 1996. The antioxidant-lipoic acid enhances insulin-stimulated glucose metabolism in insulin-resistant rat skeletal muscle. *Diabetes* 45:1024–1029.

Kakkar, Rakesh, et al. 1997. Antioxidant defense system in diabetic kidney: a time course study. *Life Sciences* 60(9):667–679.

Kao, W.H., F. Brancati, J. Nieto, et al. 1997. Serum magnesium concentration and the risk of incident NIDDM: the atherosclerosis risk in communities (ARIC) study. *Diabetes* 46(Suppl 1):20A.

Lee, N.A., and C.A. Reasner. 1994. Beneficial effect of chromium supplementation on serum triglyceride levels in NIDDM. *Diabetes Care* 17:1449–1452.

Mukherjee, B., S. Anbazhaga, A. Roy, et al. 1998. Novel implications of the potential role of selenium on antioxidant status in streptozotocin-induced diabetic mice. *Biomedicine and Pharmacotherapy* 52:89–95.

Osterode, W., et al. 1996. Nutritional antioxidants, red cell membrane fluidity and blood viscosity in type I (insulin dependent) diabetes mellitus. *Diabetic Medicine* 13:1044–1050.

Paolisso, G., S. Sgambato, A. Gambardella, et al. 1992. Daily magnesium supplements improve glucose handling in elderly subjects. *American Journal of Clinical Nutrition* 55:1161–1167.

Preuss, H.G., S.T. Jarrell, R. Scheckenbach, et al. 1998. Comparative effects of chromium, vanadium and Gymnema sylvestre on sugar-induced blood pressure elevations in SHR. *Journal of the American College of Nutrition* 17:116–123.

Rett, K., M. Wicklmayr, P. Ruus, et al. 1996. Alpha-liponsaure (thioactsäure) steigert die insulinempfindlichkeit übergewichtiger patienten mit type-II-diabetes. *Diabetes und Stoffwechsel* 5(suppl 3):59–62.

Shanmugasundaram, E.R.B. 1990. Possible regeneration of the islets of Langerhans in streptozotocin-diabetic rats given Gymnema sylvestre leaf extracts. *Journal of Ethnopharmacology* 30:265–279.

Sharma R.D., T.C. Raghuram, and N.S. Rao. 1990. Effect of fenugreek seeds on blood glucose and serum lipids in type I diabetes. *European Journal of Clinical Nutrition* 44:301–306.

Singh, R.B., A.N. Mohammed,S.S. Rastogi, et al. 1998. Current zinc intake and risk of diabetes and coronary artery disease and factors associated with insulin resistance in rural and urban populations of north India. *Journal of the American College of Nutrition* 17:564–570.

Trehan, Shruti, et al. 1996. Magnesium disorders: what to do when homeostasis goes awry. *Consultant* 1996:2485–2497.

Vaccaro, Olga, et al. 1997. Moderate hyperhomocysteinaemia and retinopathy in insulin-dependent diabetes. *Lance* 349:1102–1103.

Zeyuan, D., T. Bingvin T., and L. Xiaolin. 1998. Effect of green tea and black tea on the blood glucose, the blood triglyceride, and antioxidation in aged rats. *Journal of Agricultural and Food Chemistry* 46:3875–3878.

Chapter Eleven

American Diabetes Association. 2000. Position statement: diabetes mellitus and exercise. *Clinical Practice Recommendations* 23 (Suppl 1).

Durak, Erik P. 1998. *Exercise and Diabetes: A Guidebook for Health Professionals*, published through Medical Health and Fitness. Santa Barbara, California.

Galbo, H., J. J. Holst, and N. J. Christensen. 1979. The effect of different diets of insulin on the hormonal response to prolonged exercise. *Acta Physiology Scandinavia* 107:19–32.

Kern, P. A., J. M. Ong, B. Soffan, and J. Catty. 1990. The effects of weight loss on the activity and expression of adipose-tissue lipoprotein lipase in very obese individuals. *New England Journal of Medicine* 322:1053–1059.

Schneider, S.H., et al. 1992. Ten year experience with an exercise-based outpatient lifestyle modification program in the therapy of diabetes mellitus. *Diabetes Care* 15(suppl):1800–10.

Tuominen, J.A., et al. 1997. Exercise increases insulin clearance in healthy men and insulin-dependent diabetes mellitus patients. *Clinical Physiology* 17:19–30.

Turner, R., et al. 1996. UK prospective diabetes study – 17: a 9-year update of a randomized, controlled trial of improved metabolic control on complications in non-insulin-dependent diabetes mellitus. *Annals of Internal Medicine* 124(1 pt 2):136–45.

www.drearlmindell.com

Visit Dr. Mindell's website to check his speaking and radio schedule, read his blog, sign up for his newsletter, and find out what his latest favorite supplements and books are!

www.virginiahopkinstestkits.com

Visit Virginia Hopkins' website for reader-friendly information about prescription alternatives, natural remedies, drug warnings, and bioidentical hormones, and sign up for her newsletter.

More Books by Dr. Earl Mindell and Virginia Hopkins

Prescription Alternatives 4th Edition: Hundreds of Safe, Natural, Prescription-Free Remedies to Restore & Maintain Your Health,
Earl Mindell, RPh, PhD and Virginia Hopkins

Earl Mindell's New Vitamin Bible
Earl Mindell, RPh, PhD and Hester Mundis

What Your Doctor May Not Tell You about Menopause
John R. Lee, MD and Virginia Hopkins

Dr. John Lee's Hormone Balance Made Simple
John R. Lee, MD and Virginia Hopkins

ABOUT THE AUTHORS

Earl Mindell, RPh, PhD, is the best selling author of *Earl Mindell's Vitamin Bible*, which has sold more than 10,000,000 copies worldwide. Dr. Mindell is a registered pharmacist, a master herbalist, and a professor of nutrition at Pacific Western University in Los Angeles. He conducts nutrition seminars around the world.

He is the author or co-author of over 30 books, including:

Earl Mindell's New Vitamin Bible

Earl Mindell's New Herb Bible

Prescription Alternatives

Earl Mindell's Supplement Bible

The MSM Miracle

Dr. Earl Mindell's Natural Remedies

Dr. Earl Mindell's Nutrition and Health for Dogs

Parents' Nutrition Bible

Earl Mindell's Food as Medicine

Earl Mindell's Soy Miracle

The Anti-ageing Bible

Arthritis Miracle

Dr. Earl Mindell's Secrets of Natural Health

Dr. Mindell provides nutritional information and free assessments at www.drearlmindell.com.

Virginia Hopkins, M.A., has been a writer and editor since she graduated from Yale University in 1976. She has a master's degree in Applied Psychology from the University of Santa Monica.

Virginia is the co-author, with John R. Lee, M.D. of the books:

Dr. John Lee's Hormone Balance Made Simple

What Your Doctor May Not Tell You About Breast Cancer

What Your Doctor May Not Tell You About Premenopause

And the best-selling classic, *What Your Doctor May Not Tell You About Menopause*

Virginia was the managing editor of "The John R. Lee, M.D. Medical Letter" and has or co-authored and/or ghost written more than 30 books on alternative health and nutrition. She is currently the editor of the "Virginia Hopkins Health Watch," an e-mail newsletter with a wide readership which can be viewed at www. virginiahopkinstestkits.com.